PARTNERING FOR RECOVERY IN MENTAL HEALTH

PARTNERING FOR RECOVERY IN MENTAL HEALTH

A PRACTICAL GUIDE TO PERSON-CENTERED PLANNING

Janis Tondora, Psy.D.

Assistant Professor, Department of Psychiatry
Yale University School of Medicine, New Haven, CT

Rebecca Miller, Ph.D.

Associate Research Scientist, Department of Psychiatry
Yale University School of Medicine, New Haven, CT

Mike Slade Ph.D.

Professor of Health Services Research
Health Service and Population Research Department,
Institute of Psychiatry King's College London, London, UK

Larry Davidson, Ph.D.

Professor of Psychiatry, Department of Psychiatry
Yale University School of Medicine, New Haven, CT

WILEY

This edition first published 2014
© 2014 by John Wiley & Sons Ltd

Registered office: John Wiley & Sons, Ltd, The Atrium, Southern Gate, Chichester, West Sussex, PO19 8SQ, UK

Editorial offices: 9600 Garsington Road, Oxford, OX4 2DQ, UK
111 River Street, Hoboken, NJ 07030-5774, USA

For details of our global editorial offices, for customer services and for information about how to apply for permission to reuse the copyright material in this book please see our website at www.wiley.com/wiley-blackwell.

Library of Congress Cataloging-in-Publication Data

Symanski-Tondora, Janis L. (Janis Lee), 1971- author.
  Partnering for recovery in mental health : a practical guide to person-centered planning / Janis Tondora, Rebecca Miller, Mike Slade, Larry Davidson.–Second edition.
      p. ; cm.
  Includes bibliographical references and index.
  ISBN 978-1-118-38857-0 (pbk.)
  I. Miller, Rebecca, 1974- author. II. Slade, Mike, author. III. Davidson, Larry, author. IV. Title.
  [DNLM: 1. Mental Disorders–rehabilitation. 2. Mental Health Services. 3. Patient Care Planning–organization & administration. 4. Patient Care Team–organization & administration. 5. Patient-Centered Care–methods. WM 400]
  RC489.M53
  616.89′1–dc23

                                                                                                      2014000626

A catalogue record for this book is available from the British Library.

Wiley also publishes its books in a variety of electronic formats. Some content that appears in print may not be available in electronic books.

Cover image: iStockphoto © 4774344sean
              iStockphoto © Xavier Arnau

Set in 10/12pt TimesLTStd by Laserwords Private Limited, Chennai, India

Printed in the UK

To our children,

Caleb and Rylee

Cecilia

Emily and Isabel

and

Abbey, Alana, and Lexi

in the hope that all mental health services will be encouraging, person-centered, and collaborative if and when they, or their children, decide to use them.

Contents

Acknowledgments

This book is the result of over a decade of on-the-ground development, implementation, and evaluation of a person-centered approach to recovery planning for adults with serious mental illnesses. Consequently, there are far too many individuals who have been instrumental in this process for us to acknowledge each and every one of the service users, clinical practitioners, peer staff, family members, administrators, system leaders, and advocates by name. Nonetheless, we thank you all for your invaluable contributions to this work. We think that you know who you are.

Without diminishing the importance of the collective wisdom of our various collaborators, we do want to single out a number of individuals and organizations that have either made this work possible or made it as effective as it is. The first stages of this work were supported by a grant from the US National Institute of Mental Health (NIMH) to Davidson and a contract with the US Substance Abuse and Mental Health Services Administration (SAMHSA) to Tondora to work with a talented group of people to develop an early version of a person-centered care manual. For their contributions to this work, we thank Diane Grieder, Steve Onken, Sade Ali, Neal Adams, Linda Rammler, and Rita Cronise. Diane and Neal are also to be thanked for their tireless efforts to promote dialog around person-centered planning internationally and for Diane, in particular, for her partnership and contributions to our many shared training and consultation efforts these past several years.

Subsequently, our evolving work benefitted from the steadfast interest and energetic support of two Commissioners of the State of Connecticut's Department of Mental Health and Addiction Services, Thomas Kirk, Jr., and Patricia Rehmer. With their financial and moral commitment to implementing person-centered care planning across the state system, we were able to secure additional funding from both SAMHSA and the US Centers for Medicare and Medicaid Services to further refine and evaluate this approach. Most recently, we received additional support from the NIMH to evaluate implementation in Delaware and Texas, and we extend our thanks to our colleagues in those states as well. Finally, sabbaticals for both Davidson and Slade from Yale and King's College, respectively, have provided the much needed reviewing and writing time to help bring this manual to completion.

In the following chapters, we make the point that it is not "person-centered" to insist that a person make his own decisions when his cultural and personal preference is for a more collective decision-making process involving family members, elders, or other respected parties. We also point out that it is not in keeping with the principles of "person first language" to insist that a person describe herself as a "woman with an addiction" when she prefers to use the term "addict" (even though that may be offensive to others). These are but two examples of the ways in which we have seen well-meaning practitioners turn person-centered principles on their head in the earnest attempt to be faithful to what they interpret person-centeredness to be. We offer this manual in the hope that readers will feel as free to "fiddle" with aspects of this approach as they may need to be faithful to it, and that above all, being person-centered means respecting the uniqueness and honoring the dignity of each individual you have the privilege to serve.

Janis Tondora, Psy.D.
Yale University School of Medicine

Rebecca Miller, Ph.D.
Yale University School of Medicine

Mike Slade Ph.D.
Institute of Psychiatry King's College London

Larry Davidson, Ph.D.
Yale University School of Medicine

Module 1: What is mental health recovery and how does it relate to person-centered care planning?

Goal

This module introduces the key concepts in mental health recovery and recovery-oriented practice. It reviews the history and development of "person-centered" care planning and places it within the broader context of recovery-oriented efforts that are transforming the mental health system as a whole.

Learning Objectives

After completing this module, you will be better able to:

- define mental health recovery;
- describe the difference between traditional practices and recovery-oriented approaches;
- define person-centered care planning;
- understand how person-centered planning differs from past practice.

Learning Assessment

A learning assessment is included at the end of the module. If you are already familiar with mental health recovery and its implications for care planning, you can go to the end of this module to take the assessment section to test your understanding.

Recovery is about living a fulfilling and rewarding life in the context of mental health challenges. While some people recover in the sense that they no longer experience psychiatric symptoms, recovery is not necessarily about becoming symptom- or problem-free. A large part of recovery for many people is moving beyond being labeled as a "mental patient,"

Partnering for Recovery in Mental Health: A Practical Guide to Person-Centered Planning, First Edition.
Janis Tondora, Rebecca Miller, Mike Slade and Larry Davidson.
© 2014 John Wiley & Sons, Ltd. Published 2014 by John Wiley & Sons, Ltd.

"client," or even "consumer" to find new meaning, purpose, and possibility in life. For many people, recovery means [1]:

- No longer defining oneself by the experience of mental illness.
- Being a full participant in the community with valued roles such as worker, parent, student, neighbor, friend, artist, tenant, lover, and citizen.
- Running one's own life and making one's own decisions.
- Having a rich network of personal and social support outside of the mental health system.
- Celebrating the newfound strength and skills gained from living with, and recovering from, mental illness.
- Having hope and optimism for the future.

> *R*ecovery is a journey of healing and transformation enabling a person with a mental health problem to live a meaningful life in a community of his or her choice while striving to achieve his or her full potential.
>
> —*SAMHSA National Consensus Statement on Mental Health Recovery* [2]

All around the world people have been demonstrating the possibility, and reality, of mental health recovery. Their stories of lived experience are supported by a mounting evidence base that suggests that recovery is more the norm than the exception in serious mental illness. Beginning with the World Health Organization's (WHO) International Pilot Study of Schizophrenia launched in 1967, there have been a series of long-term, longitudinal studies conducted that have produced a consistent picture of broad heterogeneity in outcome for persons with serious mental illnesses. For example, with respect to schizophrenia, the WHO study documented partial to full recovery in between 45% and 65% of each sample, even when recovery was defined in a clinical fashion as a remission in symptoms, while an even larger percentage of people were able to live independently despite continued symptoms [3].

Similarly, the Vermont Longitudinal Study conducted by Courtney Harding and colleagues found recovery or significant improvement in 62%–68% of the people studied—a finding that was all the more important given that the research was carried out on individuals discharged from a state hospital who were considered to have the most severe and persistent of conditions [4]. Since then, eight more long-term studies (e.g., 22–37 years) have been completed around the world, yielding comparable—and at times, better—results [5].

The evidence for the prevalence of recovery and the potential for recovery-oriented care to help people live full lives has recently been gathered in two landmark texts published by the Boston University Center for Psychiatric Rehabilitation [6]. These books present a summary of over 30 years of experience that challenges the long-held view that serious mental illnesses typically follow a deteriorating course, and explore the range of interventions that have been employed to promote recovery for persons with these conditions.[1] Readers seeking a briefer overview of the

> *R*ecovery is a process, a way of life, an attitude, and a way of approaching the day's challenges… The need is to meet the challenge of the disability and to re-establish a new and valued sense of integrity and purpose within and beyond the limits of the disability; the aspiration is to live, work, and love in a community in which one makes a significant contribution.
>
> —*Deegan* [7]

---

[1] For more information, see: www.bu.edu/cpr/products/books/titles/rsmi-2.html.

empirical evidence for recovery in serious mental illness are referred to an essay on this topic by Ed Knight, Vice President of Recovery, Rehabilitation, and Mutual Support for Value Options.[2]

Where Did the Idea of Mental Health Recovery Come From?

The idea that people can—and do—actually recover from serious mental illnesses grew in large part from the personal experiences and stories of people who experienced recovery in their own lives. Their voices and perspectives were diverse and were from people who were receiving mental health services ("users" of services); individuals who believed they had survived despite the treatment they received ("psychiatric survivors"); and people who had once been patients receiving services, but who felt they had moved beyond that status in their lives and were now "ex-patients." These voices provide the most powerful, and persuasive, testament to recovery, and readers who are interested in reading such stories can find them in websites such as www.SAMHSA.gov/Recoverytopractice (from the United States), www.recoverydevon.co.uk (from England) and www.scottishrecovery.net (from Scotland), to name a few.

These voices and perspectives merged to form a movement that has not only survived, but has also grown and emerged as a powerful force for change in mental health policy and services around the world. Drawing on personal experiences, social justice values, civil and human rights, and a passion for changing the mental health system, users/survivors have been the driving force behind the recovery movement that promises to significantly impact both public policy and treatment practices around the globe [8].

> *R*ecovery is a process by which an individual with a disability recovers self-esteem, dreams, self worth, pride, choice, dignity, and meaning.
>
> —*Townsend & Glassner* [9]

Is Mental Health Recovery the Same as Recovery from Addiction?

A variety of self-help and 12-step programs in the addictions arena has influenced the recovery movement and the value it places on mutual support and shared experience. However, there are some unique differences between the actual experience of recovery in mental illness as compared to recovery from addiction. For example, there are core differences related to issues of power. A common requirement in 12-step programs is to admit powerlessness and turn one's self and life over to a "Higher Power." While respecting the importance spirituality plays in many people's lives, mental health recovery emphasizes empowerment and

---

[2] This document is available at: http://csipmh.rfmh.org/Knight_recovery.htm.

self-determination as well; helping individuals to find their own voice and to take personal responsibility for their own lives. This is based on the belief that people need to reclaim, not turn over, their power as one of the first steps of recovery.

This distinction between mental health and addiction recovery impacts both the process of self-identification and the use of preferred language and terms. For example, traditional 12-step programs encourage individuals to introduce themselves as: "My name is X and I am an alcoholic." This is consistent with the 12-step focus on acknowledging one's powerlessness over a substance, and self-identification in this manner is respected as a part of the individual's unique recovery process. In contrast, in the mental health recovery community, there is an emphasis on helping individuals to move beyond the diagnostic labels that have been applied to them by others. Therefore, individuals are encouraged to use "person-first" language and thereby NOT to identify themselves, or allow themselves to be identified by others, in any way that makes a psychiatric diagnosis their most salient or defining characteristic: for example, "My name is X and I am schizophrenic." In both the addiction and mental health contexts, it is important to note that individual preferences around language and self-identification vary widely, and additional guidance on this topic is offered in Module 2.

Despite these differences in the process of recovery in mental illness and addiction, there are numerous areas of overlap and commonality [10]. The important thing to remember is that no matter what an individual's particular label or diagnosis, people with mental illnesses and addictions are first and foremost people, and people who know best what kind of life they will find worth living in the wake of a behavioral health condition. This is the hallmark of the recovery movement in both mental health and addiction.

Getting Beyond Us versus Them

When we say that "people with mental illnesses and addictions are first and foremost people," we mean that "they" are fundamentally the same as "us" (i.e., those persons who do not have a mental illness or addiction). Though we may be stating the obvious when we say that people with mental illnesses are still people, the reality and experiences in the past have suggested otherwise. Consider Table 1.1. On the left are the things we typically consider to be important in leading a satisfying life, while on the right are the things that have traditionally been identified in care plans as important for persons with serious mental illnesses. 1) What differences do you see in the lists below? 2) What are the similarities? and 3) Are there differences in tone and language between the two lists?

People receiving mental health services want essentially the same things out of life that practitioners do—a home, family, faith, a sense of purpose, health, and other such things. As a result, "recovery" for mental health service users should involve pretty much the same things that mental health service practitioners see as being a part of their own well-being and quality of life. Yet systems are structured in such a way that practitioners are seldom prompted to think of it in this manner. This is particularly true in the context of service planning where "compliance" (with treatment, administering of medications, program rules, etc.) is by far the most commonly identified desired outcome in the "what we expect for them" list reflected in written treatment plans. Recovery-oriented and person-centered care is, at its core, about getting past this "us/them" dynamic to truly partner with people in recovery in their efforts to attain their personally defined and valued goals.

Table 1.1 "Us and Them"

What We Expect for "Us"	What We Expect for "Them"
✓ A life worth living	✓ Attends program, groups, clubhouses
✓ A home to call my own	✓ Residential stability
✓ Faith, spiritual connections	✓ Better judgment
✓ A real job, financial independence	✓ Decreased symptoms/stability
✓ Being a good spouse … parent	✓ Increased insight … accepts illness
✓ Friends	✓ Decreased hospitalization
✓ Joy, fun	✓ Compliance
✓ Nature	✓ Abstinence
✓ Music	✓ Increased functioning
✓ Love … intimacy … sex	✓ Cognitive functioning
✓ Learning, growing	✓ Realistic expectations

Recovery as an Emerging Global Paradigm

A number of prominent reports reflect the emergence of recovery and recovery-oriented care as the driving force behind mental health systems across the globe. For example, a 2012 issue of the *International Review of Psychiatry* contained papers outlining the current stage of recovery research and practice from Austria, Australia, Canada, England, Hong Kong, Israel, New Zealand, Scotland, and the United States [11], while a 2011 review of policy developments identified 30 government documents mandating recovery-oriented care from English-speaking countries around the globe [12]. The following are a few examples from these English-speaking nations:

Achieving the Promise: Transforming Mental Health Care in America, US Department of Health and Human Services [13]. This report called for recovery to be the "common, recognized outcome of mental health services" and recommended "fundamentally reforming how mental health care is delivered in America" to be reoriented to the goal of recovery. This report strongly criticized the nation's current mental health system as one that, too often, "simply manages symptoms and accepts long-term disability."

Improving the Quality of Health Care for Mental and Substance Use Conditions, Institute of Medicine [14]. This report speaks specifically of the decision-making abilities of individuals who have a mental illness as well as those who do not. One harmful stereotype that is referenced in the report is "incompetent decision making." One key recommendation notes that "to promote patient-centered care, all parties involved in health care for mental or substance use conditions should support the decision-making abilities and preferences for treatment and recovery of persons with mental and substance use problems and illnesses."

No Health without Mental Health, UK Department of Health [15]. This national policy framework for England identifies six priorities for the mental health system, including "more people will have good mental health," "more people with mental health problems will recover," and "fewer people will experience stigma and discrimination." One national initiative being carried out as part of this policy is the Implementing Recovery–Organisational Change (ImROC) program, which is working with 33 of the 55 mental health trusts (provider organizations) in England to support their transformation to a recovery orientation [16]. This initiative includes the recommendation that the mental health workforce comprise 50% people with lived experience of mental illness [17] and introduce Recovery Colleges to provide support to people with mental illnesses through an educational approach [18].

Changing Directions, Changing Lives, Mental Health Commission of Canada [19]. An emerging vehicle of change in several countries has been the establishment of influential Mental Health Commissions. The Canadian commission was established in 2007, and in developing its national mental health strategy, it has taken testimony from thousands of people living with mental health conditions. An important stepping stone was the 2009 discussion document *Toward Recovery and Well-Being* [20], which defined mental health as "*a state of well-being in which the individual realizes his or her own potential, can cope with the normal stresses of life, can work productively and fruitfully, and is able to make a contribution to her or his own community.*" In this report, a mental health framework is developed as a blueprint for change, with the strategic direction to "*foster recovery and well-being for people of all ages living with mental health problems and illnesses, and to uphold their rights.*" The emphasis on well-being in the context of mental illness is consistent with empirical research [21] and the links between well-being research and recovery are becoming clearer [22].

A Recovery Approach within the Irish Mental Health Services—A Framework for Development, Mental Health Commission of Ireland [23]. The Mental Health Commission in Ireland has created a framework for developing services across the island of Ireland, which involves a focus on the strengths and opportunities rather than the limitations and symptoms of illness. The contribution of mental health systems is understood to involve "*enabling and empowering the person to access their inner strengths and resources to build a meaningful, valued, and satisfying life.*" One transformation component that is highlighted is that of dynamic leadership because "*if the predominant ethos is one of benign paternalism and illness orientation, or one that ignores the input of service users at management and service development level, then a culture that ignores the principles of recovery is likely to be fostered throughout the organization. Equally, without a stated commitment to the principle of individualism and choice, people may simply re-title current practice as recovery-oriented.*" This focus on the role of organizational commitment is consistent with best practices internationally [11].

Blueprint II: Improving Mental Health and Well-Being for All New Zealanders, Mental Health Commission of New Zealand [24]. In 1998, New Zealand developed the first national blueprint for transformation toward recovery. In 2012, it issued a new 10-year national strategy based on the learning from Blueprint I, and addressed specifically the impact of the global economic downturn. It adopted the "Triple Aim" model as a framework for sustainable service development: 1) improving quality, safety, and experience of care; 2) improving health and equity for all populations; and 3) ensuring the best value in public health system resources. In identifying eight priority areas for service development, a shift from Blueprint 1 was evident, involving a greater focus on well-being and a more explicit reference to issues of risk and safety.

Framework for Recovery-Oriented Practice, Department of Health, Victoria [25]. Although a state-based policy rather than a national policy, this framework draws on the best available evidence internationally to identify the key domains of recovery-oriented practice:

promoting a culture of hope; encouraging autonomy and self-determination; fostering collaborative partnerships and meaningful engagement; focusing on strengths; striving for holistic and personalized care; involving family, carers, supporting people, and significant others; maximizing community participation and citizenship; showing responsiveness to diversity; and committing to ongoing reflection and learning. For each domain, the key capabilities and examples of both good practice and good leadership are provided. This is a brief and easily accessible document that informs the development of a recovery orientation as mandated in the fourth National Mental Health Plan (2009–2014) in Australia.

Cross-Cutting Principles, US Substance Abuse and Mental Health Services Administration (SAMHSA) [26]. This report establishes a set of cross-cutting principles to guide the program, policy, and resource allocation based on the belief that people of all ages, with or at risk for mental health or substance use disorders, should have the opportunity for a fulfilling life that includes an education, a job, a home, and meaningful relationships with family and friends. To further this agenda, SAMHSA put forth a *Consensus Statement* that outlines 10 fundamental components of mental health recovery as guideposts for recovery-oriented service providers, policymakers, and advocates. The consensus definition was developed through deliberations at a conference in December 2004 of over 110 expert panelists representing mental health consumers, families, providers, advocates, researchers, managed care organizations, state and local public officials, and others. These fundamental components are summarized in Table 1.2.

A Common Misconception: Is Recovery = Cure?

The widespread misinterpretation that "recovery equals cure" has generated concerns among service users, practitioners, family members, and policymakers alike who fear that recovery-oriented care will "leave certain people behind." However, the notion of mental health recovery, as defined by SAMHSA and presented in these modules, does not advocate complete symptom remission. Rather, it is personally defined and accessible to all. It involves a redefinition of one's illness as only one aspect of a multidimensional sense of self who is capable of identifying, choosing, and pursuing meaningful goals despite the effects of the illness or possible side effects of treatment or stigma.

> "*The goal of the recovery process is not to become 'normal.' The goal is to embrace our human vocation of becoming more deeply, more fully human.*
> *The goal is not normalization.*
> *The goal is to become the unique, awesome, never to be repeated human being that we are called to be.*"
>
> —Deegan [27]

In this sense, the notion of recovery borrows from the disability rights movement that argues that the elimination of the disability is not the ultimate goal. The goal is to live life to its fullest even in the face of continued limitations, for example, a person with paraplegia does not have to regain his or her mobility to have a satisfying life in the community, nor does an individual with schizophrenia have to stop hearing voices to work, worship, or volunteer. Recovery restores a positive sense of identity despite one's disability and its limitations, and it is a lifelong process that involves an indefinite number of incremental steps in various life domains.

Table 1.2   Ten Core Components of Mental Health Recovery

Self-Direction: Individuals lead, control, exercise choice over, and determine their own path of recovery by optimizing autonomy, independence, and control of resources to achieve a self-determined life.	Strengths-Based: Recovery focuses on valuing and building on the multiple capacities, resiliencies, talents, coping abilities, and inherent worth of individuals.
Individualized and Person-Centered: There are multiple pathways to recovery based on an individual's unique strengths and resiliencies as well as his or her needs, preferences, experiences (including past trauma), and cultural background in all of its diverse representations.	Peer Support: Mutual support—including the sharing of experiential knowledge and skills and social learning—can play an invaluable role in recovery.
Empowerment: Individuals have the authority to choose from a range of options and to participate in all decisions—including the allocation of resources—that will affect their lives, and are educated and supported in so doing.	Respect: Community, systems, and societal acceptance and appreciation of individuals with mental illnesses—including protecting their rights and eliminating discrimination and stigma—are crucial in achieving recovery.
Holistic: Recovery encompasses an individual's whole life, including mind, body, spirit, and community.	Responsibility: Individuals with mental illnesses have a personal responsibility for their own self-care and journey of recovery.
Nonlinear: Recovery is not a step-by-step process but one based on continual growth, occasional setbacks, and learning from experience.	Hope: Recovery provides the essential and motivating message of a better future—that individuals can and do overcome the barriers and obstacles that confront them.

(Adapted from U.S. Department of Health and Human Services, 2006).

How Does the Concept of Recovery Transform Care?

The concept of recovery is increasingly recognized as stimulating a new way to think about serious mental health problems, treatment, and outcomes, and it is gradually being accepted and incorporated by traditional mental health programs. Many practitioners are looking for new ways to relate to, and work with, people who receive services in the hope that they can transform their programs to be more recovery focused in meaningful and significant ways [7]. Often, the first step in this process is acknowledging the core differences between traditional models of care and recovery-oriented approaches.

Until fairly recently, most mental health services have been organized around a deficit-based model that perceives mental illness as a disease that must be "cured" [28] through the remission or elimination of symptoms. Because they are trained to focus on treating deficits and symptoms—the things that are wrong with people—practitioners and service delivery organizations have had a tendency to overlook the things that are right with people, such as strengths and competencies [29]. A recovery orientation shifts the focus to "the glass as half full." It is a perspective that allows us to see that no matter how disabled, "all people have existing strengths and capabilities as well as the capacity to become more competent" [30].

With all this attention on strengths, how then, does a recovery-oriented system view the very real, and sometimes serious, difficulties experienced by people living with mental illnesses? Furthermore, with its emphasis on self-determination, what does the recovery model say about the role of practitioners and clinical care?

"Both/And" rather than "Either/Or"

The notion of recovery-oriented care presented throughout this manual does not imply that exclusive power is turned over to the service user with disregard for the knowledge and value of practitioners. Rather, recovery-oriented care, and the representative practice of person-centered care planning, is based on a foundation of partnership in which there is mutual respect between the practitioner and the individual service user. While the emphasis is on maximizing the person's autonomy, the recovery paradigm also respects the expertise of the caregiver and recognizes the important role of the practitioner in the person-centered partnership.

It is equally important to acknowledge that there have been major advances made within the context of traditional clinical and rehabilitative care. Now more than ever, the mental health field has the ability to offer individuals a wider range of evidence-based practices, diagnostically based treatment modalities, and diverse medication options, and these advances have had a significant

> *Hope is a frame of mind that colors every perception. By expanding the realm of the possible, hope lays the groundwork for healing to begin.*
>
> —Jacobson & Greenley [31]

impact on the treatment of symptoms for persons with serious mental illnesses. However, no matter how skilled the professional community has become in treating the *illness*, the voice of the recovery community suggests that doing so is not sufficient in and of itself to recover the *person*—or more accurately, for the person *to recover*. The interventions of traditional clinical models will definitely continue to play an important role in transformed mental health systems, and recovery-oriented care is based on an understanding that the field can, and must, do better to reframe the goal of treatment as helping people to move beyond achieving clinical stability to recovering lives worth living. This is the essence both of recovery-oriented care planning and of recovery-oriented practice.

Hope as the Foundation

So, how will the field get there? Self-determination, freedom of choice, control over one's own life, personal responsibility, and meaningful community belonging—this is the recovery vision of a transformed mental health system. Throughout the remainder of these modules, the reader will be introduced to a wide range of strategies and tools that will assist him or her in implementing the potential recovery-oriented practice of "person-centered care planning." Yet the most essential tool that a direct care provider has at his or her disposal is the belief in the possibility of recovery for all people.

Hope is at the heart of recovery. Just as the person must hold onto hope in the journey of recovery, the practitioner must hold onto hope that recovery-oriented systems change is both possible and powerful. This belief is at the foundation of each of the modules that follow.

How Does Person-Centered Care Planning Relate to Recovery?

Person-centered care planning (PCCP) and recovery-oriented care are inherently interwoven. One cannot exist without the other. A recovery-oriented system cannot be fully realized in the absence of PCCP. PCCP is one tool that systems can use to move away from an illness-based model of diagnosis and treatment delivered by experts toward a recovery-based model of growth and achievement in which every person involved has an important role to play.

Similarly, PCCP cannot be fully implemented in the absence of a recovery-oriented culture. PCCP must be embedded in a system that is committed to changing not only what people *do* (e.g., in the practice of PCCP) but also how people *think* and *believe* about recovery and their obligation to partner with people to achieve it. PCCP is best thought of as one essential tool that should be combined with other efforts to promote system change, including such things as the expansion of peer-operated services or the modification of outcomes-monitoring plans. PCCP represents a window of opportunity to move from theory to practice and to apply the concepts and values of recovery-oriented care to prompt real and meaningful changes in care planning.

In understanding this relationship between PCCP and recovery-oriented care, it can be helpful to think of PCCP as requiring attention to the four essential "Ps" (see Figure 1.1), which are philosophy, process, plan, and product.

- **Philosophy:** the overall philosophy of the organization and the extent to which it is recovery-oriented and supports PCCP.
- **Process:** the typical planning process and whether it involves the type of collaborative interactions that are consistent with PCCP.
- **Plan:** the design of the plan itself, that is, the paper (or electronic) document, and whether it reflects a meaningful roadmap to support the person's recovery.
- **Product:** the expected outcomes associated with PCCP, that is, how an agency determines if the plan has been successful in terms that are meaningful to the persons being served and their loved ones.

> *I*n a transformed mental health system, a diagnosis of a serious mental illness ... will set in motion a well-planned, coordinated array of services and treatments defined in a single plan of care ...
> The plan will include treatment, supports, and other assistance to enable consumers to better integrate into their communities and to allow consumers to realize improved mental health and quality of life.
>
> —Final Report of the US New Freedom Commission on Mental Health [12]

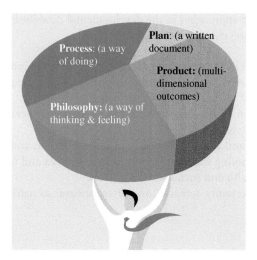

Figure 1.1   The "4 Ps" of Person-Centered Care Planning

What Does Person-Centered Care Planning Mean and Why Is It Important?

For people receiving mental health services, person-centered care means they have choices in the services they use. It means they can be an active partner in selecting their recovery support team and in inviting family members and other "natural supporters" (such as employers, tutors, neighbors) to be involved. It means realizing—or being helped to realize—that they have the power to change their lives and can partner with their recovery team in doing so. For practitioners, PCCP means partnering with people receiving services to help them achieve goals that are personally meaningful to them, even when such goals extend beyond those areas traditionally addressed by clinical care. Such goals may include returning to work, finishing school, making friends, having a girlfriend/boyfriend, or developing a hobby.

PCCP as presented in these modules is informed by many sources, particularly the experiences of people who have "survived" the limitations of traditional models of care to call for radical change toward more person-centered planning. In addition, the vision of PCCP in the mental health field is informed by similar efforts in other disability fields. For example, some of the earliest and most prominent "person-centered planning" models were developed in the 1980s by professionals and advocates in the developmental disabilities field. These include

- Whole-life planning [32]
- Lifestyle planning [33]
- McGill Action Planning System [34]
- Personal futures planning [35]

Although each of these approaches in the developmental disabilities field varies somewhat, they all share the following characteristics [36]:

- The primary direction in the planning process comes from the individual, or his or her family or designated other when the person is under age or incapacitated and the family or other is empowered to speak on his or her behalf.
- Maximum involvement of significant others and a reliance on personal relationships as a primary source of support.
- A focus on capacities and assets rather than on just limitations and deficits.
- An emphasis on promoting the use of community resources and nonsegregated settings outside the formal health and social service systems.
- An acceptance of uncertainty, setbacks, and disagreements as natural steps on the path to self-determination.

Is This Really any Different from Traditional Approaches to Care Planning?

Traditional models of care planning are often referred to as deficit or illness-based models. These models differ across setting and service providers but can generally be characterized as follows:

- Attention is paid primarily to illnesses, symptoms, or impairments.
- Emphasis is on eradicating or managing illness rather than specifically promoting recovery.
- Role of person with mental illness is often passive and limited to following the practitioner's recommendations or suggestions, such as taking medications and "avoiding stress".
- Perhaps most importantly, community inclusion and personal choice are viewed as rewards that follow from successful treatment (i.e., you will be able to live by yourself and return to school once you take your medication consistently and your symptoms are stable), rather than as basic human and civil rights that provide the foundation for the person's efforts toward recovery.

Some of the limitations of these traditional models include the following:

- Power is allocated largely (or only) to the service provider to determine diagnosis and to develop treatment goals.
- People receiving services are not commonly encouraged to take an active or self-directed role, which fosters both short-term disengagement and long-term institutional dependency.
- Service agencies focus on systemically defined outcomes (e.g., hospitalization rates) and are held less accountable for other outcomes that hold real value for those they serve (e.g., employment, relationships, community activities).
- Success is most often determined by system standards and is gauged on narrowly defined goals such as treatment compliance or symptom reduction.

- Services are typically fragmented and disconnected from other important parts of a person's life. For example, mental health services are typically provided separate and apart from primary health care. Another example of service fragmentation is the lack of connection between the mental health system and a spiritual or faith community.

Treatment planning practices delivered within more traditional models are heavily influenced by these limitations:

- Traditional treatment planning is seen as more of a peripheral and bureaucratic paperwork task rather than as a central focus of the recovery-oriented relationship.
- Planning meetings are still sometimes carried out in the absence of the person served. When individuals receiving services are present, their role is generally limited and often involves simply signing the plan to acknowledge that he or she "participated" in the process, with little or no attention paid to whether or not that "participation" was substantive or meaningful.
- Treatment "teams" typically consist of a variety of paid mental health service providers with minimal, if any, direct involvement of natural supporters such as family and friends (assuming such involvement is desired by the individual).
- Traditional treatment plans respond to individuals' needs largely through a reliance on specialized services designed for persons with a label of mental illness rather than through a focus on community inclusion and resources. For example, a service user who identified bowling or reading as a desired activity might be encouraged to initiate bowling outings from the local psychosocial clubhouse or start a reading group there rather than join a bowling league or a neighborhood book club that is already taking place in the community.
- Treatment goals are often based on the person receiving services demonstrating an expected level of engagement in treatment, for example, medication or treatment compliance. Failure to meet such goals may then be attributed to the person's lack of "motivation" rather than the system's failure to deliver person-centered services or other factors such as a person's choice, or lack of resources.

Status of PCCP Implementation

Despite the limitations of traditional treatment planning models, person-centered care planning (PCCP) has not yet been widely accepted or adopted by the mental health system—particularly in contrast to person-centered planning as implemented in the developmental disabilities service system [37]. There are many reasons for this, but some can be found in understanding that PCCP is:

- Not widely taught in professional or graduate training programs.
- Viewed as an administrative burden and an exercise in paperwork.
- Not valued as a clinical intervention or as a means to build a therapeutic alliance.
- Seen as a "risky business" because of a belief that allowing service users choices and self-determination in their own care could lead to poor decision making and disastrous consequences.

- Viewed as not something that people in the process of recovery are interested in.
- Viewed as somehow inconsistent with the clinical rigor expected in the process and documentation by funders (e.g., Centers for Medicare and Medicaid Services) and accreditors (e.g., Joint Commission on Accreditation of Healthcare Organizations).

But for those mental health practitioners and organizations that have fully embraced recovery and person-centered practices, the co-created care plan becomes:

- An essential part of services.
- A strategy for managing complexity.
- An opportunity for collaborative and creative thinking.
- An opportunity to thoughtfully support individuals in taking next steps, trying new activities, and expanding natural support networks.
- Something that is valued, by service user and practitioner alike, as a meaningful roadmap to recovery.
- A tool for gauging progress toward valued short and long-term recovery goals.

Table 1.3. summarizes the contrasts between a recovery-oriented and a person-centered approach as compared with a more traditional treatment approach. Module 2 will provide greater detail regarding the translation of each of these principles into the *practices* of person-centered care planning.

What Does PCCP *Actually Look Like* in Practice?

While much greater detail regarding both the *process* and *documentation* of PCCP will be shared in subsequent modules, we conclude this module with an example that previews how a person-centered plan might look very different in practice. This scenario is based on an actual case consultation with a treatment team that requested support in developing a rigorous person-centered plan for someone we will call "Mr. Gonzalez." Mr. Gonzalez was initially described by the team as having "limited insight regarding his mental health and addictions issues," which led to "frequent refusal to take meds and to participate in treatment." Below is a snapshot of his story.

> *Mr. Gonzalez, a 31-year-old married Puerto Rican man, is living with bipolar disorder and a co-occurring addiction to alcohol that he often uses to manage distressing symptoms. During a recent period of acute mania, Mr. Gonzalez had increasingly volatile arguments with his wife in the presence of his two young sons. On one such occasion, he pushed his wife across the room that prompted her to call the police. When the police arrived, Mr. Gonzalez was initially uncooperative and upset. After he calmed down, Mrs. Gonzalez agreed not to press charges, but insisted her husband leave the house and meet with his clinician the following morning.*

Table 1.3 Summary of Contrast between Traditional and Person-Centered Approaches to Service Planning

Traditional Approaches	Person-Centered Approach
Self-determination comes after individuals have successfully achieved clinical stability	Self-determination and community inclusion are viewed as fundamental human rights of all people
Compliance is valued	Active participation and empowerment are valued
Largely one-directional; clearly delineated professional boundaries	Reciprocity in relationship; engaged, collaborative relationship
Jargon and reductionist terms and labels common	Strengths and respect-based communication in written/spoken language
Only professionals have access to information (e.g., plans, assessments, records)	All parties have full access to the same information—often referred to as "transparency."
Symptoms, disabilities, and deficits drive treatment; targeted professional solutions	Plans capitalize on strengths and the value of life experiences
Lower expectations	Higher expectations
Facility-based settings and professional supporters	Integrated settings and natural/community supports are seen as crucial
Avoidance of risk; protection of person and community	Acceptance of the dignity of risk and a focus on growth
Clinical stability or managing illness	Achievement of broad-based life goals
Lack of individualization; "cookie-cutter" service design	Cultural preferences and values more actively incorporated in individualized care
Assumptions regarding readiness/desire for active treatment	Sensitivity to stage of change; meeting people "where they are at"

Mr. Gonzalez's wife is actively involved in his recovery and treatment, and she is open to reconciliation. However, she made it clear that he would not be allowed to live at home, or visit with his sons, until he "gets control of himself." Upon visiting the Community Mental Health Center the following morning, Mr. Gonzalez tells his clinician repeatedly that his love for his family and his faith in God are the only things that keep him going when things are rough and he does not know what he will do without them. More than anything, he wants to be able to reunite with his family and be a good role model for his sons. He feels that the only person who understands this is the Center Peer Specialist with whom he has a close relationship.

A few weeks after the incidents described here, the treatment team contacted us and requested consultation, as they were clearly frustrated with Mr. Gonzalez. They noted that he had "great potential" but was "refusing to meet them half way." Prior to meeting with the team and Mr. Gonzalez, we requested that a copy of the working treatment plan be shared with us so that we could get familiar with the story. A look at the treatment plan made it clear that the plan had been drafted with limited, if any, substantive input from Mr. Gonzalez, with a focus on four narrowly defined clinical problem areas.

The numbered goals on "his" treatment plan included achieving and maintaining clinical stability; reducing assaultive behavior; complying with medications; and achieving abstinence. These goals were then followed by objectives related to such things as attending scheduled groups; taking meds as prescribed; demonstrating insight into illness; submitting to urine toxicology screens, and so on. This is not to say that all these things are necessarily negative or undesirable. However, they do not, in and of themselves, equate with the realization of Mr. Gonzalez's valued long-term recovery goals! Nor do they reflect any respect for Mr. Gonzalez as a *unique* human being. Mr. Gonzalez's working treatment plan could have just as easily been for Mr. Smith, Mr. Reyes, or Mr. Martino as there was virtually NO mention of his personal recovery goals. It is critical that the treatment plan not be completely divorced from that which is most valued by, and motivating to, the individual—in the case of Mr. Gonzalez, his love for his family, his desire for reconciliation, and his wish to be "a better role model" to his boys.

When presented with this feedback, the treatment team began to see that their style of working with Mr. Gonzalez might, in fact, have been one of the factors leading to the very disengagement and "noncompliance" that had generated their request for consultation in the first place. To what extent could they really expect him to actively work a recovery plan that he had no part in creating—a plan that had little, if any, connection to his most valued goals and priorities? Given this, it is not surprising that Mr. Gonzalez was reluctant to talk to the doctor about his lithium, to attend the "anger-management" group, or to show up for his toxicology screens. What had been attributed initially to the "patient's noncompliance and denial" was, in fact, far more complicated and driven, at least in part, by the team's inability to really listen to, and understand, Mr. Gonzalez, and to reflect that in a collaboratively developed recovery plan.

Now let us shift to a discussion on how Mr. Gonalez's care plan might look different through the lens of recovery-oriented, person-centered care. First and foremost, the plan should begin with, and be driven by, the priority goals as stated by Mr. Gonzalez. Next, it should reflect the strengths and resources that may be particularly significant in achieving his current goals. This is then balanced by a clear statement of the clinical and/or psychosocial issues that may be interfering with progress. These barriers should be acknowledged alongside his assets and strengths, as this is essential in maintaining clinical rigor in the documentation, providing targeted and effective interventions, and justifying the "medical necessity" of treatment. Next, the plan should include short-term objectives that reflect desired concrete changes in behavior or functioning that are meaningful to Mr. Gonzalez. And, finally, a quality person-centered care plan should conclude with a mix of services and action steps (carried out by practitioners, natural supporters, and the person him/herself) that help Mr. Gonzalez to overcome barriers and move forward in his personal recovery journey.

Each of these points is discussed in greater detail in subsequent modules, but for now we leave you with a graphic representation that illustrates how PCCP departs from traditional practice by integrating Mr. Gonzalez's strengths, preferences, and valued goals in a

A Traditional Treatment Plan

Goal(s):

- *Achieve and maintain clinical stability*
- *Reduce assultive behavior*
- *Comply with medications*
- *Achieve abstinence*

Objective(s):

- Pt will attend all scheduled groups; pt will meet with psychiatrist and take all meds as prescribed; pt will complete anger management program; pt will demonstrate increased insight re: clinical symptoms; pt will recognize role of substances in exacerbating aggressive behavior.

Services:

- Psychiatrist will provide medication management 1x/mos. for 3 mos. to stabilize symptoms; Rehab specialist will provide Anger Management Group 1x/wk for 6 weeks; Nursing staff will monitor medication compliance; Psychologist will provide individual therapy 2x/mo for purpose of increasing insight into bipolar illness; Addictions Counselor will conduct random tox screens to monitor abstinence.

Toward Person-Centered Planning

Life Goal:
I want to get my family back and be a good father to my boys.

Strengths to Draw Upon:	Barriers Which Interfere:
Devoted father; motivated for change; supportive wife; faith & prayer are source of strength/comfort; connected to Peer Specialist	Acute symptoms led to arguments/aggression in the home; lack of coping strategies; abuse of alcohol escalates behavioral problems

Sample Short-Term Objective

Within 30 days, Mr. Gonzalez will use learned coping strategies to have a minimum of two successful visits with wife & children as reported by Mrs. Gonzalez in family therapy session.

Services & Supports

-M.D. to provide med management 2x/mo for 3 mos. to reduce irritability & distressing symptoms.

-Clinician to provide weekly family therapy sessions for one mos. for purpose of discussing Mrs. Gonzalez's expectations and to negotiate a possible family reunification plan.

-Rehab Specialist to provide Communication and Coping Skills Training 1x/wk. for 1 mos. to coach/practice skills which will support successful visits with wife and children.

-Center Chaplain will meet with Mr. Gonzalez 2x/mo. to promote use of faith/daily prayer as positive coping strategy to manage distress.

-Center Peer Specialist will provide weekly Wellness Recovery Action Plan group to promote daily wellness through use of self-directed strategies.

Figure 1.2   From Traditional Planning to Person-Centered Care Planning

person-centered care plan that simultaneously respects the role of high quality mental health services. More than simply a rewritten treatment plan, this process represented a dramatic shift in the very nature of the relationship between Mr. Gonzalez and his treatment team. They shared a commitment to co-create a more hopeful recovery vision for the future and a practical plan for how all would work together to achieve it. No longer feeling excluded and depersonalized, Mr. Gonzalez (the formerly labeled "noncompliant patient") gradually developed a sense of trust in his team and began to actively participate in, and benefit from, the care he had previously rejected as he worked toward reuniting with his family. Together, Mr. Gonzalez and his team learned that person-centered planning was both possible and powerful (Figure 1.2).

Exercises

Exercise 1. Consider the following questions

1. How are the 10 components of recovery described above reflected in your agency and the services you deliver?
2. What are your strengths as an agency?
3. What are the areas in need of improvement?
4. How do you think service users would respond to this question?
5. How do you think they experience getting help?
6. In what ways are the services in your agency organized around symptoms? In what ways are they organized to promote recovery?
7. What changes in the provision of service does your organization need to make to move toward a person-directed, recovery-oriented system?
8. How might the quote "The goal of the recovery process is not to become 'normal' … " impact the clinical policy and practice within your organization?
9. How might the international reports in this module help you as an administrator or supervisor to change mental health care practices within your organization?
10. What would your biggest fears be regarding reorganizing your service delivery system to become recovery-oriented?
11. Looking into the future, if the vision of recovery-oriented care is realized, how will your organization be different? What will services look like when a person walks through the front door?
12. Do most of the direct care staff in your organization think that recovery is possible for everyone with a mental illness? Have you assessed recovery attitudes and beliefs among the staff members? If so, how?
13. What can be done to help support team members to be more comfortable with the idea that recovery is possible for everyone no matter what s/he looks like today?
14. Do the individuals you support believe recovery is possible for them? How can you and/or your staff engage service users to "believe" in their own recovery? How can this be built into care on a practical level?
15. The implementation of person-centered planning requires attention to each of the four "Ps". Which areas are the most challenging for you/your organization? Which areas represent strengths to build upon?

Exercise 2. *What If …?*

1. Write down three things that are important to you in your life, the things that give you meaning, keep you happy or healthy, or are reasons that you get up in the morning.
   - Now count up and down each item until you reach 7, and cross off that item.
2. How did it feel to cross off that item? How did that feel to imagine your life without those things?
3. How does this relate to the experience of treatment planning? Can you think of examples in traditional treatment planning where important things are "crossed off" of peoples' lists?

Take home message:

Traditional treatment has involved other people having the power to decide the focus of a service user's care over the next 3–6 months—what makes it on the list and what doesn't. Think of situations in which people are told they cannot be supported in moving out of the group home until they have been medication compliant for six months, or cannot be referred to a supported employment program to get a job until they have done "90 meetings in 90 days." People in recovery report that this experience feels like others "crossing off" deeply valued goals from their personal list, such as moving into a home of one's own or securing a job to feel proud of.

- Some service users are excluded completely from these decisions, others are told it is "not in their best interest" or the "timing is not right" to … go back to school or to work … to move out of the group home … to regain custody of their children, and so on.
- Most treatment plans continue to identify the goals of clinical stability, compliance with medications, and abstinence from drugs and alcohol as the highest priorities—to the exclusion of other life domains that are critical elements of anyone's sense of well-being.
- In developing a plan for recovery, remember this exercise and how it feels to have something important to you crossed off your list … said it was not a priority … said you needed to wait….

Now imagine what your attitude and response to this kind of treatment would be if this were not just an exercise … What if?

Learning Assessment

Module 1: What is mental health recovery and how does it relate to person-centered care planning?		
Statement	True	False
1. Recovery requires the reduction or remission of symptoms of mental illness.		
2. The pursuit of community activities and valued roles is important for recovery.		
3. Traditional mental health care is mainly focused on identifying and addressing deficits.		
4. Adherence to psychiatric medications is a necessary prerequisite for recovery.		
5. The goal of recovery is to become normal.		
See the Answer Key at the end of the chapter for correct answers. **Number Correct**		
0 to 2: Don't be discouraged. Learning is an ongoing process! You can review the Module for greater knowledge. 3 to 4: You have a solid foundation. Use this Module to enhance your skills. 5: You are ahead of the game! Use this Module to teach others and strive for excellence!		

References

1. Leamy, M., Bird, V., Le Boutillier, C., Williams, J., & Slade, M. (2011). Conceptual framework for personal recovery in mental health: systematic review and narrative Synthesis. *The British Journal of Psychiatry*, **199**, 445–451.
2. Department of Health and Human Services. (2006) *National Consensus Statement on Mental Health Recovery*. Substance Abuse and Mental Health Services Administration, Rockville, MD.
3. Jablensky A, Sartorius N, Ernberg G *et al.* (1992) Schizophrenia: Manifestations, incidence and course in different cultures. A World Health Organization ten-country study. *Psychological Medicine*, Monograph Supplement **20**.
4. Harding CM, Brooks GW, Ashikaga T *et al.* (1987) The Vermont longitudinal study, II: Long-term outcome of subjects who once met the criteria for DSM-III schizophrenia. *American Journal of Psychiatry* **144**, 727–735.
5. Slade M, Amering M, Oades L. (2008) Recovery: an international perspective. *Epidemiologia e Psichiatria Sociale* **17**, 128–137.
6. Davidson L, Harding CM, Spaniol L. (eds.) (2005, 2006) *Recovery from Severe Mental Illnesses: Research Evidence and Implications for Practice*, Volumes I-II. Center for Psychiatric Rehabilitation, Boston University, Boston.

7. Deegan, PE. (1988) Recovery: The lived experience of rehabilitation. *Psychosocial Rehabilitation Journal* **2**, 11–19.
8. Chamberlin J. (1990). The Ex-Patients' Movement: Where we've been and where we're going. *The Journal of Mind and Behavior* **11**, 323–336.
9. Townsend W, Glassner N. (2003) Recovery: the heart and soul of treatment. *Psychiatric Rehabilitation Journal* **27**, 83–86.
10. Davidson L, White W. (2007) The concept of recovery as an organizing principle for integrating mental health and addiction services. *Journal of Behavioral Health Services and Research* **34**, 109–120.
11. Slade M, Adams N, O'Hagan M. (2012). Recovery: past progress and future challenges. *International Review of Psychiatry* **24**, 1–4.
12. Le Boutillier C, Leamy M, Bird VJ *et al.* (2011) What does recovery mean in practice? A qualitative analysis of international recovery-oriented practice guidance. *Psychiatric Services* **62**, 1470–1476.
13. Department of Health and Human Services. (2003) *Achieving the Promise: Transforming Mental Health Care in America.* Substance Abuse and Mental Health Services Administration, Rockville, MD.
14. Institute of Medicine. (2005) *Committee on Crossing the Quality Chasm: Adaptation to Mental Health and Addictive Disorders.* The National Academies Press, Washington, DC.
15. Department of Health. (2011) *No Health without Mental Health.* Department of Health, London.
16. ImROC Team. (2012) *Supporting Recovery in Mental Health.* NHS Confederation, London.
17. Shepherd G, Boardman J, Burns M. (2010) *Implementing Recovery. A methodology for organisation change.* Sainsbury Centre for Mental Health, London.
18. Perkins R, Repper J, Rinaldi M *et al.* (2012) *ImROC Briefing Paper 1: Recovery Colleges.* NHS Confederation, London.
19. Mental Health Commission of Canada. (2012) *Changing Directions, Changing Lives.* Mental Health Commission of Canada, Ottawa, ON.
20. Mental Health Commission of Canada. (2009). *Toward Recovery and Well-Being.* Mental Health Commission of Canada, Ottawa, ON.
21. Keyes CLM. (2005) Mental illness and/or mental health? Investigating axioms of the complete state model of health. *Journal of Consulting and Clinical Psychology* **73**, 539–548.
22. Slade M. (2010) Mental illness and well-being: The central importance of positive psychology and recovery approaches. *BMC Health Services Research* **10**, 26.
23. Mental Health Commission of Ireland. (2008) *A Recovery Approach within the Irish Mental Health Services – A Framework for Development.* Mental Health Commission, Dublin.
24. Mental Health Commission of New Zealand. (2012) *Blueprint II: Improving Mental Health and Wellbeing for all New Zealanders.* Mental Health Commission, Wellington, NZ.
25. Department of Health in Victoria. (2011) *Framework for Recovery-Oriented Practice.* Department of Health, Melbourne.
26. SAMHSA. (2004) *Cross-Cutting Principles.* Substance Abuse and Mental Health Services Administration, Rockville, MD.

27. Deegan PE. (1996) Recovery as a journey of the heart. *Psychiatric Rehabilitation Journal* **19**, 91–97.
28. Corrigan PW, Penn DL. (1999) Lessons from social psychology on discrediting psychiatric stigma. *American Psychologist* **54**, 765–776.
29. Davidson L, Strauss JS. (1995) Beyond the biopsychosocial model: Integrating disorder, health and recovery. *Psychiatry: Interpersonal and Biological Processes* **58**, 44–55.
30. Grills C, Bass K, Brown DL *et al.* (1999) Empowerment evaluation: Building upon a tradition of activism in the African American community. In: Fetterman DM, Kaftarian SJ & Wandersman A (eds.) *Empowerment evaluation: Knowledge and tools for self-assessment and accountability.* Sage Publications, Thousand Oaks, CA.
31. Jacobson N, Greenley D. (2001) What is recovery? A conceptual model and explication. *Psychiatric Services* **52**, 482–485.
32. Butterworth J, Hagner H, Heikkinen B *et al.* (1993) *Whole Life Planning: A Guide for Organizers and Facilitators.* Training and Research Institute for People with Disabilities, Boston, MA.
33. O'Brien J. (1987) A guide to life-style planning: Using the activities catalog to integrate services and natural support systems. In: Wilcox B & Bellamy GT (eds.) *A comprehensive guide to the activities catalog.* Paul Brookes, Baltimore, MD.
34. Vandercook T, York J, Forest M. (1989) The McGill Action Planning System (MAPS): A strategy for building the future. *Journal of the Association of Persons with Severe Handicaps* **14**, 205–215.
35. Mount B, Zwernik K. (1988) *It's Never too Early; It's Never too Late: A Booklet about Personal Futures Planning.* Metropolitan Council, St. Paul, MN.
36. O'Brien J, Lovett H. (1992). *Finding A Way Toward Everyday Lives: The Contribution of Person Centered Planning.* Pennsylvania Department of Mental Retardation, Harrisburg, PA.
37. O'Brien C, O'Brien J. (2000) *The Origins of Person-Centered Planning: A Community of Practice Perspective.* Responsive Systems Associates, Syracuse, NY.

Answers to the Learning Assessment:

1. F
2. T
3. T
4. F
5. F

Module 2: Key principles and practices of person-centered care planning

Goal

This module introduces the fundamental values of person-centered care planning (PCCP) and describes how each translates into practice. Of particular importance is the development of an engaged and trusting relationship within which the practitioner can explore different ways of co-creating plans in partnership with persons in recovery.

Learning Objectives

After completing this module, you will be better able to:

- discuss the values and principles of person-centered care planning;
- appreciate the importance of engaging persons in recovery in trusting and collaborative partnerships as the necessary foundation for recovery planning;
- identify the key practices of person-centered care planning across multiple domains.

Learning Assessment

A learning assessment is included at the end of this module. If you are already familiar with the subject of person-centered care planning, go test your knowledge. Then you can focus your learning efforts on the material that is new for you.

A Caveat[1]

A cautionary note is necessary prior to presenting details regarding the principles and practices of person-centered care planning (PCCP). PCCP cannot be carried out as though it

[1] (Adapted from Tondora and colleagues [1]).

Partnering for Recovery in Mental Health: A Practical Guide to Person-Centered Planning, First Edition.
Janis Tondora, Rebecca Miller, Mike Slade and Larry Davidson.
© 2014 John Wiley & Sons, Ltd. Published 2014 by John Wiley & Sons, Ltd.

were some straightforward or simple thing like inserting "Tab A" into "Slot B." The emphasis on the "nuts and bolts" in this module, and those that follow, should by no means be taken to suggest such an approach. In fact, such a rigid adherence to a single model or a set of standards would be antithetical to the core premises of PCCP.

Nonetheless, there are several strategies that illustrate what PCCP is and what it is not. These are articulated to offer guidance (not directives) for well-intended practitioners who ask the question—as they so often do—"What can we do differently *today* when we sit down with Tisha to assure that her plan is truly person-centered?"

This being said, it is important to recognize that each organization, each local community, and each country is different—with a range of clinical traditions and standards, regulations, funding strategies, and so on. The intent of this module is NOT to endorse one standardized model or way of doing things. Rather, reflective practices are reviewed in an effort, in the words of O'Brien [2], to "encourage the flowering of diverse methods … that express the many different gifts of those people who accept responsibility for the work," and responsibility to walk beside and support people on their unique paths to recovery and wellness. Practitioners are encouraged to incorporate the strategies, tools, and suggestions offered in the remainder of this text in the manner that best suits the abilities, needs, and preferences of the people they serve.

Key Principles and Practices of PCCP

The following section elaborates on the core principles of PCCP as introduced in Module 1. Each of the principles is grounded in an appreciation that PCCP is, at its core, about respecting an individual's human rights to participate fully in community life in a self-determined way. Key practices within PCCP are also identified to highlight how these more abstract concepts can be translated into real and meaningful changes in mental health service settings. Though some practices certainly

> *T*he question of planning ownership—or "who owns the plan?"—in person-centered planning is undeniably central. Yet, as we consider this key question, it may be more enlightening to ask ourselves instead, "who owns the person's life?"
>
> —Jonikas and colleagues [3]

cut across various principles, for clarity we have included each practice a single time only in the discussion of the most relevant principle.

Self-determination and community inclusion are fundamental human rights for all people.

> No right is held more sacred, or is more carefully guarded, by the common law, than the right of every individual to the possession and control of his[/her] own person, free from all restraint or interference of others, unless by clear and unquestioned authority of law.
>
> —US Supreme Court, Union Pacific Railway Co. v. Botsford [4]

The quotes here and below highlight the fact that PCCP is based fundamentally on a civil rights model of psychiatric disability. This model views self-determination and participation in community life as basic human rights of people with mental illnesses rather than as privileges that have to be earned either through compliance with care or through the acquisition of a variety of social, cognitive, or behavioral skills.

Recovery and PCCP are built on the principle that people with mental illness do not have to successfully "complete treatment" or be cured of their illness in order to participate fully in community life. This approach has profound implications for the structure of mental health care across the globe, because achievements such as meaningful jobs, intimate relationships, and a home to call one's own are not things that come after a person has recovered. Rather, they are at the heart of the person-centered recovery process all along! In PCCP, we recognize that the person owns his or her life, and, as a result, should drive the planning process to the maximum extent possible. This assumption is not nullified by labels, noncompliance, or perceived "stage" of recovery.

Believing that treating symptoms is the first order of business (while delaying attention to broad-based life goals) can lead systems to establish a continuum of services that individuals are directed to progress through in a linear fashion. For example, it is common for referrals to vocational rehabilitation programs to be controlled by a clinical practitioner. In addition, people are often required to demonstrate "work readiness" or "symptomatic stability" as a prerequisite to entry into such programs. This means that the practitioner will sign off on the referral only when the person has "proven" that he or she is ready for employment through compliance with treatment and the demonstration of clinical stability.

> *O*wnership of one's life isn't a tangible thing that comes with a guarantee or warranty. It is a physical, mental, spiritual, and responsible connection/reconnection to life for an individual who seeks his/her own destiny.
>
> —Nancy Fudge, as quoted in Jonikas and colleagues [3]

However, abundant literature has shown that these types of screening procedures and criteria have limited predictive validity regarding success in the workplace. Requiring people to move through services in this manner also neglects the fact that activities such as working are often the path through which people become clinically stable in the first place. PCCP respects the nonlinear nature of recovery and service participation, and encourages individuals in choosing from a flexible array of supports as needed.

What does this look like in practice?

- Individuals are not required to attain, or maintain, clinical stability or abstinence before being supported by the care planning team in pursuing such goals as employment, education, or housing.
- People are encouraged to pursue their recovery in whatever "order" or nonlinear fashion they choose, with the least number of "hoops" to jump through, for example, people have direct access to recovery services (such as supported employment, supported education) rather than being subject to "gate-keeping" where the referral is controlled solely by a clinical practitioner. A preestablished continuum of services is replaced with a flexible array of supports that individuals can choose from based on their unique needs and preferences and how these might shift over time.

Active participation and empowerment is vital

Self-determination requires that individuals have the right to control the direction of their lives and their treatment free from undue external influence. This includes the right to exercise control in the planning of services and supports. In PCCP, there is an emphasis on personal empowerment and maximizing one's ability to make life-defining decisions involving one's living situation, relationships, vocation, education, and other areas of life.

All participants in the care planning process must understand, and respect, that the recovery journey belongs to the person receiving care. Practitioners may provide the person metaphorically with a car, but it is the person who must then take over and occupy the driver's seat. As with driving, the person will need to be educated about various options and their potential consequences, but he or she will be the one to *drive* the car, and, to extend the metaphor, to drive his or her own recovery plan. Active participation and empowerment of the person receiving services is vital. Participation that is limited to passive compliance is seen as potentially damaging in that it reinforces a sense of hopelessness and interferes with the activation, learning, and growth necessary for people to advance in their recovery.

Particular attention must be paid, however, to the fact that this emphasis on self-determination and autonomy in PCCP may appear to conflict with some individuals' cultural values. For example, family-centered and collective processes may be more central to goal setting and decision making in some African, Hispanic, Asian, and Native American cultures. If the individual expresses such a cultural preference or value, practitioners should manage the planning process in a way that legitimizes a more collective decision-making approach [5]. For example, when a person expresses a cultural preference to defer to a parent or a community elder in the decision-making process, the practitioner can encourage that person's participation and support him or her in taking an important and active role throughout the process. This may be achieved by the parent or elder exercising leadership directly in a planning meeting or perhaps by this person offering his or her input in a less directive fashion.

Either way, it is important to recognize that such adaptations in the decision-making process are actually consistent, rather than contradictory, with the principles of person-centered care, as it is the person himself or herself who is asked and can express his or her preferences for how decision making is to be carried out. While the process may seem to be the same on the surface, there is a world of difference between someone making decisions for an individual without their consent versus someone making decisions because the individual has, in fact, invited them to do so for whatever reasons.

Finally, it is essential that practitioners develop competency in the emerging best practice of shared decision making (SDM) if they are to support maximum self-determination in the PCCP process. SDM is relatively new in the mental health arena, and, as yet, there is no one consensus-definition of the term. However, in the widely referenced SAMHSA report *Shared Decision Making: Making Recovery Real in Mental Health* [6], SDM has been described as a way for service users and practitioners to improve communication about treatment options to arrive at more collaborative decisions that respect individuals' preferences, goals, and cultural values. In this sense, when used effectively, shared decision making is one tool practitioners can use to help put the person back at the center of person-centered care.

While the authors see SDM as an important development that supports transformation and the adoption of PCCP, SDM, in and of itself, is not sufficient for a number of reasons to realize the vision of PCCP presented in this text. First, as is the case with many emerging recovery-based approaches, the concrete practices of SDM have yet to be fully articulated in a manner that will support accountability in the field. Its hallmark decision aids, while promising, are limited in scope most often (applying specifically to *treatment* decisions) and are not yet widely available to service users or practitioners. As we have learned through years of our own PCCP consultation, in the face of ambiguity, it is not uncommon for practitioners to assert "we already do it." As applied to SDM, at best, this runs the risk of watered-down implementation, and at worst, this can result in SDM becoming a "euphemism for persuasion or pressure to consent rather than fulfilling its promise as supported self-determination" [8].

> Shared decision-making is founded on the premise that two experts are in the consultation room … neither … should be silenced, and both must share information in order to arrive at the best treatment decisions possible.
>
> —Deegan [7]

The authors caution against this and remain hopeful that SDM will be delivered in the spirit it was originally intended as it holds great potential to facilitate respectful communication and service user empowerment. However, high-quality PCCP requires that SDM NOT be offered in isolation from the multiple other diverse key practices presented throughout this text, and also that it NOT be limited to the context of *treatment* decisions but also applied to the broader arena of *life* choices that PCCP aims to uphold.

What does this look like in practice?

- An individual may select or change practitioners within agency guidelines and is aware of the procedures for doing so. If guidelines are overly restrictive, they should be revisited and potentially modified with inputs from the persons served.
- The individual is a partner in all recovery and care planning activities or meetings, except under emergency and/or extreme circumstances (which are clearly documented in the person's medical record).
- The plan is based on the goals and priorities identified by the person receiving services and, when appropriate, in conjunction with those who the person wishes to involve in the PCCP process.
- The person receiving services has reasonable control over the nature and logistics of the planning process, including invitees, the location of the care planning meeting, and the degree to which he or she wishes to make decisions autonomously or in deference to the respected others.
- Individuals are given advance notice of all planning meetings so that they can adequately prepare to participate and/or arrange to have supportive others attend.
- Practitioners develop competency in the emerging best practice of SDM. They routinely make use of the available SDM decision aids and supports, and encourage service users to do the same. For example, print workbooks, educational videos, online interactive decision aids, and other "cool tools," which are available at the SAMHSA Shared Decision Making Website www.samhsa.gov/consumersurvivor/sdm/StartHere.html

Developing trusting, reciprocal, and collaborative relationships is key

One of the key ways in which recovery-oriented care has been distinguished from traditional approaches is that it attends first and foremost to the *person* with the mental health condition, rather than, say, to the symptoms of the illness or to the diagnosis. The importance of this shift from illness or diagnosis to person permeates first-person accounts, in which people consistently identify "having someone who believed in me" as one of the most important factors in their recovery. While treatments may be useful in addressing illness, having a foundation of support in trusting, accepting relationships in which the person feels valued as a human being appears to offer a necessary basis for the person to take up "the work of recovery" [9].

While such support obviously should, and often does, come from important people in the person's life such as family and friends, first-person accounts suggest that mental health care is most effective when it involves this kind of relationship as well. This may, in part, be in reaction to the experiences of stigma and discrimination persons with mental illnesses have often encountered in mental health settings in the past, with one function of recovery-oriented care being to help the person repair the damage done by previous negative experiences. The need for mental health practitioners to engage in respectful, trusting, and collaborative relationships may also be in response to the nature of some of the damage done by the mental illnesses themselves. Above and beyond—or perhaps underneath—experiences of discrimination, the disruptions caused by the illness may further undermine a person's sense of self, making the restoration of his or her "personhood" a major focus of care early in the recovery process.

In fact, in mental health care, attending in this way first and foremost to the *person* has been a well-accepted principle of the recovery movement from its very inception. It was highlighted as early as 1992 by Pat Deegan, for example, when she suggested that "the concept of recovery is rooted in the simple yet profound realization that people who have been diagnosed with a mental illness are human beings" [11]. William Anthony [12] likewise argued that the transcendent principle of recovery is the attention it draws to the fundamental "personhood" of people with mental illnesses.

> *R*ather than subsuming the entirety of the person, a psychiatric label is but one aspect of a person who otherwise has assets, interests, aspirations, and the desire and ability to continue to be in control of his or her own life.
>
> —Connecticut Department of Mental Health and Addiction Services, Practice Guidelines for Recovery-Oriented Behavioral Health Care [10]

In order to be aligned with these principles, recovery-oriented practices—practices that are aimed at helping to restore the person's basic sense of personhood—can no longer perpetuate the neutral or abstinent stance advocated originally by Freud. Service users have described the dispassionate stance taken by many mental health practitioners as contributing to, rather than lessening, their sense of no longer being a person. One-directional relationships, in which one party does all the giving and the other party does all the taking, leaves the second party feeling diminished rather than enhanced [13]. Understanding these limitations of therapeutic abstinence has led recovery-oriented practitioners to adopt a more engaged—and still professional—stance in which a core part of their role is to validate the person's fundamental personhood and assist the person in reconstructing a self, and a life, in the wake of the illness and the effects of prejudice. As a longtime mental health consumer advocate in the United States, Ed Knight, once remarked, in order to participate in PCCP, "you first have to believe that you have the right to be a person."

Recovery-oriented practitioners convey this very important message to persons with mental illnesses by demonstrating a genuine sense of compassion and by remembering—as suggested by Deegan [14]—that, no matter what the diagnosis or the severity of the illness, the person remains a human being deserving care and love. Recovery-oriented practitioners communicate this message also by providing a safe space in which the person can feel welcomed, supported, and valued, and in which the person is invited to talk about the things that matter to him or her—whatever they may be—and in which the practitioner will take the time to listen. Perhaps most importantly, practitioners convey this message by showing common human concern for the person's everyday life. It is this concern with helping to make the person's everyday life better, despite the illness and its effects, which provides the necessary context and foundation for developing a recovery plan that has that as its primary focus.

What does this look like in practice?

- Practitioners view persons receiving services first and foremost as human beings deserving care and compassion and capable of giving it in return. Agencies examine their policies closely regarding clinical "boundaries" and how these impact the therapeutic relationship, for example, are practitioners allowed to accept gifts or tokens of appreciation as gestures of reciprocity and a person's desire to "give back?"
- Practitioners view persons receiving services as experts on their own lives, asking them what has worked/not worked in their recovery process and reflecting this input in their care plan.
- Practitioners hold and convey the hope that the person's life can be improved. Ambitious goals are not discounted as "unrealistic" but appreciated as a reflection of the person's persistence and resilience. Practitioners also share accurate, research-based information regarding the broad heterogeneity in outcomes for persons with mental illnesses rather than defaulting to assumptions of chronicity and lifelong service enrollment and dependence.
- Practitioners take an active interest in the person's everyday life, in a conversational rather than interrogational manner, and help to identify and explore ways that the person's life can be improved in ways that are important to the person. This includes openness to conversations around a person's intimate connections to other human beings and/or a spiritual higher power, that is, conversations about God and sex! Many clinical practitioners continue to be uncomfortable exploring this territory despite the fact that persons with mental illnesses often report that these relationships are at the core of their recovery.

Language matters and should reflect recovery values

Despite the fact that the process behind PCCP may be largely recovery-oriented, the translation of this process into the actual language of the document itself continues to be a core challenge to many practitioners who are committed to creating person-centered plans.

The following are offered as overarching guidelines that should be considered regarding the language that is incorporated in both the written documents and the verbal interactions in practice.

What does this look like in practice?

- Use person first and verbatim language. This avoids being either stigmatizing or objectifying. "Person first" language is used to acknowledge that the disability is not as important as the person's individuality and humanity, for example, "a person with schizophrenia" versus "a schizophrenic" or a "person with an addiction" versus "an addict." Employing person first language does not mean that a person's disability is hidden or seen as irrelevant but that it is not to be the sole focus of any description about that person. To make it the sole focus is depersonalizing and derogatory, and is no longer considered an acceptable practice.

  While the majority of people with disabilities prefer to be referred to in this manner, when in doubt, ask the individual what he or she prefers. Use of person-first language is intended to support a person's positive sense of identity apart from his or her illness. It is not intended to be seen as a superordinate principle that applies universally to all individuals. Within the 12-Step Fellowship of Alcoholics Anonymous, for example, early steps in the recovery process involve admitting one's powerlessness over a substance and acknowledging how one's life has become unmanageable. It is therefore common for such individuals to introduce themselves as "My name is X and I am an alcoholic." This kind of preference is respected as a part of the individual's unique recovery, and it is understood that it would be contrary to person-centered principles to pressure the person to identify as "a person with alcoholism" in the name of person first language.
- Efforts are made to record each individual's responses verbatim, and to use that person's words as much as possible, rather than translating the information into professional language. This helps to ensure that the plan remains narrative-based and person centered. If and when technical language must be used, it is first translated appropriately and presented in a person first, nonoffensive manner, for example, avoiding the language of "dysfunction" or "deficit." It is to be expected, for example, that more clinical components of a recovery plan will need to address what professionals currently consider to be the symptoms of the mental health condition the person has. It is more accurate and useful—as well as respectful—however, to state that the person "will hear fewer distressing voices" or "hear distressing voices less often" than to identity "reduction of auditory hallucinations" or simply "decreased symptoms" as an objective on the person's recovery plan.
- Use language that reflects a resilience framework. Practitioners work to interpret perceived deficits, difficulties, and impairments within a strength and resilience framework, identifying the person receiving services less with the limitations of the disorder and more with his or her active attempts to manage the condition. For example, an individual who takes medication irregularly may currently be perceived primarily as "noncompliant," "lacking insight," or "requiring monitoring to take meds as prescribed." These concepts are consistent with problem-centered plans. It is also possible, however, for this same individual to be perceived as "making use of alternative coping strategies such as exercise and relaxation to reduce reliance on medications" or could be praised for "working

collaboratively to develop a contingency plan for when medications are to be used on an 'as-needed' basis."

In a strengths and resilience framework, words such as "hope," "coping," and "recovery" are used frequently in the documentation and delivery of services. There are seldom, if ever, times when people are not doing anything at all on their own behalf. It has been our experience that, while it may sometimes require concerted efforts on the part of the practitioner to discern what efforts the person is making, people are much more often actively trying to find ways to deal with their life situation. When this is not easily seen in any given individual's case, practitioners are encouraged to remember the following explanation offered by Pat Deegan, who herself had experienced such periods of apparent passivity and withdrawal:

> The professionals called it apathy and lack of motivation. They blamed it on our illness. But they don't understand that giving up is a highly motivated and goal-directed behavior. For us, giving up was a way of surviving. Giving up, refusing to hope, not trying, not caring; all of these were ways of trying to protect the last fragile traces of our spirit and our selfhood from undergoing another crushing [15].

- Use descriptive language whenever possible. Avoid using diagnostic labels as "catch-all" means of describing an individual (e.g., "Is a 22-year-old borderline patient with ... "), as such labels tend to be deficit-oriented and they often yield minimal information regarding the person's actual experience or manifestation of illness. Alternatively, an individual's needs are best captured by an accurate description of his or her strengths and limitations. For example, the term "low-functioning" is commonly found in records, yet this term offers little by way of informing a meaningful rehabilitation intervention. This is not to suggest that an individual's struggles are discounted. However, it is far more useful to provide a description of exactly how a person's symptoms interfere with completing the daily activities and pursuing valued recovery goals. While diagnostic terms may be required for other purposes (e.g., classifying the individual to receive reimbursement from funders), their use should be limited elsewhere in the PCCP document and replaced with a descriptive focus on how the symptoms impact the person's life.
- Use empowering language. The language used also can be empowering, avoiding the eliciting of pity or sympathy, as this can cast people with disabilities in a passive "victim" role and reinforce negative stereotypes. For example, just as we have learned to refer to "people who use wheelchairs" as opposed to "the wheelchair bound," we should refer to "individuals who use medication as a recovery tool" as opposed to people who are "dependent on medication for clinical stability."

There are many terms that have been used to refer to individuals who experience mental illness including person in recovery, person with a mental illness, person labeled with a psychiatric disorder, mental health consumer or service user, person with a psychiatric disability, and so on. With the exception of the adherence to "person first" language principles, there is little conceptual agreement regarding the preferred or most appropriate terminology. In many cases, it is appropriate to speak simply to the "person," and to use terms such as individual, person in recovery, person seeking services, and so on, as we try to do in this text. However, alternative terms may be utilized depending on the context and the function of the communication. For example, "consumer" or "service user" may be used to reflect the language that has been incorporated in prominent government reports and is frequently endorsed by advocacy organizations, while a "person with a psychiatric disability" may be used to underscore the sociopolitical and civil rights dimensions of recovery-oriented care and person-centered planning.

All parties have full access to the same information

In a PCCP process, the person (and family as relevant) is provided with support and information before the planning meeting so that they can be prepared and participate as equals (e.g., [16]). Equal access to information, often referred to as *transparency*, is essential to level the playing field and to allow all parties involved to participate as valued members of the team and the planning process. Transparency also means that people can see their records at any time; since they are offered a copy of their recovery plan, they can write in their record to express alternative views or augment what has already been written. In addition, records should be readily available so that when new situations arise, wheels are not reinvented and the person and his/her team can learn from past experiences.

> Automatically offering a written copy of the recovery plan to the service user and inviting his/her review and feedback is considered an essential practice in PCCP. For example, "We met last week with the Team to talk about your priorities over the next few months and I've taken a stab at drafting the recovery plan—along with the goals, objectives, and interventions we discussed in the meeting. I'd like to take a few minutes and go over this with you to make sure we got it right. And I'd also like you to keep a copy for your records because the plan is going to be an important tool that helps shape how we work together moving forward." Offering a copy of the plan, and being open to feedback and revisions, is consistent with the notion of transparency in the relationship as the plan itself is an important manifestation of the partnership on which PCCP is based. In addition, this key practice—perhaps more so than many other strategies—can have a simple, yet powerful impact on your PCCP implementation. Knowing ahead of time that you will be placing a written copy of the plan in the individual's hands and supporting him or her in reviewing it and offering a feedback often improves dramatically the quality of the written document as practitioners will find they are sensitized to the type of language they use in describing the person and his/her life while also working diligently to really honor the person's preferences and priorities in the drafting of the plan content.

> *Transparency means plans are written, to the extent possible, using the person's own words and all parties have access to the same information in order to embrace and effectively carry out responsibilities associated with the recovery plan and process*
>
> —Osher and Osher [17]

What does this look like in practice?

- Language used in the plan is understandable to all, and when there is jargon, terms are explained to all involved.

- The person receiving services is ALWAYS offered a copy of the plan and is given an opportunity to provide the feedback. Offering a copy of the plan is an important reflection of the partnership on which the plan is based and it sends a message that the plan is an important part of the process and not just a "paperwork" requirement to satisfy the medical record.

Plans capitalize on the strengths and the value of lived experience

PCCP values and builds on the multiple capacities, resiliencies, talents, coping abilities, and the inherent worth of the individuals. The strengths and needs of the person are stated from the person's own perspective, and planning makes use of what they already know works in their own life. This may include things that may not necessarily be valued in the mainstream or dominant culture. For example, a person may see spirituality as a strength even though the time spent cultivating this might make it difficult for him or her to obtain employment. In this respect, it is useful to recall D. W. Winnicott's conclusion that "with human beings, there is an infinite variety in normality or health" [18]. It is not for the practitioner to determine how a person *should* spend his or her time. It is rather for the person himself or herself to identify those activities or pursuits that he or she "has reason to value" [19].

What does this look in practice?

- All care planning is based on a strength-based assessment in order to identify abilities and supports in the process. This assessment focuses on all life domains including those that may not be covered in equal measure by traditional psychiatric intake or interview instruments. See Module 4 for further explanation and guidance on partnering in the development of a strength-based assessment.
- Strengths are identified and incorporated as an integral part of the plan and a key element in the recovery process.
- Illness self-management strategies and daily wellness approaches such as Wellness Recovery Action Planning [20] are respected as highly effective, person-directed recovery tools, and are fully explored in the strengths-based assessment process.

> *T*here is this little pub down the street that I just love. I like to go there and have a tonic and lime and just chat with the patrons. I am not sure what it is about that place?? But it makes me feel good. Maybe ... maybe it's a lot like 'Cheers'—you know, a place where everybody knows my name ... I am just Gerry, period. Not "Gerry the mental patient ... "
>
> —Connecticut Department of Mental Health and Addiction Services, Practice Guidelines for Recovery-Oriented Behavioral Health Care [10]

High expectations for recovery are the norm

The vision of person-centered planning and self-determination is, and should remain, the pursuit of an ambitious ideal but one that is, ironically, based simply on the attainment of goals that are universal to typical human experiences—goals which appreciate our common humanity, our common aspirations and dreams, and our common sense of responsibility to become contributing members of society. Setting the bar high means focusing on choice and control; valued and enduring relationships; freedom, health, and safety and decent places to live; economic security; opportunities for community membership and contribution; and support by nurturing and caring human service professionals.

—Nerney [21]

Outcomes for people with mental illnesses need to include the expectations and aspirations shared by all humans, not just lower-order thresholds or standards commonly valued in the human service system (e.g., stability, compliance, satisfaction with services). High expectations should be the norm for all people and not reserved only for those who are judged by practitioners to have reached a certain stage or phase of recovery. As described in the quote from Nerney, at the level of everyday life, most of us want the same kinds of things. Valued, enduring relationships, opportunities for community membership, and economic security are reasonable expectations for everyone, no matter how severe or disabling a condition one may have.

What does this look like in practice?

- Not defaulting to "stability" goals and objectives, but instead working with the person in a concerted manner to discover something in his or her life that he or she would like to see change or be better.
- Setting goals and creating objectives that emerge from the person's hopes and dreams. Goal statements are not discounted as "unrealistic" but are seen as a reflection of ambitious expectations for recovery and an opportunity to inspire hope (even if such goals may need to be broken down into much smaller, modest objectives).
- Creating objectives that set the bar high, but also are agreed upon by the person and his or her care team as something that is within reach in a reasonable amount of time.
- Objectives change over time, reflecting changing expectations and circumstances. Often times plans can be recycled over several months or years, without reflection upon what is and is not working, and adjustment to the size of steps has to be done. An objective that isn't reached can be an opportunity to discuss what did happen, what went awry, and what might be a different approach to support the desired change. This works as well to continue to inspire hope, as an unmet objective is used as a chance to brainstorm and regroup, and not to punish or shame.

Natural community activities and relationships are emphasized

Recovery-oriented systems respect the fact that services and professionals should not remain central to a person's life over time. For this reason, person-centered plans recognize the value of building natural community connections as an antidote to potential lifelong dependency on formal mental health services.

PCCP supports access to inclusive community settings while seeking to reduce, or eliminate altogether, the time spent in segregated settings designed solely to support people diagnosed with a mental illness. It should be stated, however, that this focus on promoting access to integrated settings should not preclude a person from participating in activities or programs alongside other individuals with mental illnesses when such participation represents an informed choice that is a source of *positive* collective identity and pride—such as what may be found within consumer-survivor advocacy organizations, peer-run centers, or psychosocial club-

> *T*raditional mental health systems have been described as tending to surround people with serious mental health problems with a sea of professionally delivered services... which stigmatize them and set them apart from the community
>
> —Nelson and colleagues [22]

houses. This would be an example where participation in the activity or program designed solely for persons with mental illnesses is a freely chosen personal decision rather than one that is based on a restricted range of options and/or a belief that one cannot, or would not, be welcome in a more integrated setting.

The important thing to keep in mind is that while specialized service settings can play a pivotal role in an individual's recovery, over prolonged periods of time they can also tend to perpetuate a sense of chronic alienation (or "patient-hood") while also perpetuating discriminatory and unethical practices on the part of community members. For example, it was common in the past for mental health systems to offer sheltered workshops rather than real jobs for real pay in real communities. Even today, well-intended agencies continue to host movie nights at the mental health center rather than negotiating free passes to the local theater; provide internal GED classes rather than consulting with local Adult Education departments to improve their accessibility; or offer a range of facility-based spirituality groups rather than building bridges with local faith-based communities. Just as meaningful community life is not what comes *after* recovery, it is also not something that service systems can, or should, create *for* people in artificial microcosms. While these efforts to provide recreational, health-based, spiritual, and other diverse services are well-intended and represent one type of valued option within a range of services, these should not be offered to the exclusion of efforts to build pathways to more integrated community life—something we have come to refer to as the "trap of the one stop shop."

Research has highlighted the detrimental effects of the one-stop-shop and noted that local mental health systems—no matter how integrated and coordinated—cannot fully and effectively support recovery in isolation from the broader community [23–25]. For people with mental illnesses to move beyond the confines of a formal system of services and supports (what has been called the *new backward* in the community), avenues of access to regular activities in natural settings need to be opened up and supported [26]. This understanding supports recent advances in psychiatric rehabilitation that aim to help people attain or regain regular social roles such as a tenant, student, or employee within the broader community. This shift is consistent with the desires of people in recovery who express a strong preference to live in typical housing, to have friendships and intimate relationships with a wide range of people, to work in regular employment settings, and to participate in school, worship, recreation, shopping, and other pursuits alongside fellow (nondisabled) community members [27].

Care planning, at the outset, during, and in times of transition, must therefore shift from a focus on "fixing" individual deficits to an asset-based perspective that sees individual recovery as taking place in the context of a matrix of community activities and natural support relationships. Building these connections and supports becomes a priority for the care planning team as a cornerstone of the person's sustained recovery. Establishing such connections *in vivo*, in natural community settings, is a core component of recovery-oriented psychiatric rehabilitation and is essential in improving outcomes in the various domains targeted (e.g., secure housing, academic achievement, competitive employment).

The *in vivo* approach of teaching and supporting skills in the community may not replace altogether, but rather enhance, those skill development opportunities that are currently available in mental health systems. For example, many individuals benefit from the opportunity to apply both social and daily living skills in programs in which they are surrounded, and supported by, a community of recovering people. However, the added incorporation of an *in vivo* approach is necessary to capitalize on this experience and transfer skills to a more natural environment. Research on the lack of behavioral skills generalization beyond the context of formal "skills classes" (e.g., [28]) suggests that skills should be learned, and taught, to the maximum extent possible, in the context of relationships and activities that occur naturally within the larger community where those skills are actually required.

Finally, just as it is important to support people in looking outward and maximizing participation in community activities, it is equally critical to consider the value of inviting natural supporters into the PCCP process. If it is the person's preference, it can be particularly useful to include such individuals in the team, as they often have critical input and encouragement to offer. Natural supporters are people such as family members, friends, acquaintances, coworkers, fellow churchgoers, and others who are not paid to be in the person's life but who choose to be because of their personal connection to the individual or family. A diverse team, including both professional and natural supporters, is more likely to be able to think creatively to define and access supports, including supports never before conceived but necessary for recovery to occur. Just as no one ever thought of hand controls for people who could not use their legs in driving a car until one person envisioned them, so too do we need to creatively develop recovery supports when what is currently available is insufficient.

> *W*hen he asked me: "So how can I best be of help!" I thought, "Oh great, I've really got a green one. You are supposed to be the professional—you tell me!" But I get it now. I need to decide what I need to move ahead in my recovery. And I needed to know it was OK to ask people for that. That was the key.
>
> —Connecticut Department of Mental Health and Addiction Services Practice Guidelines for Recovery-Oriented Care for Mental Health and Substance Use Conditions [10]

In summary, interventions and supports should complement, rather than interfere with, what people are already doing to keep themselves well and this includes drawing strengths from community-based resources as well as diverse natural support networks. These should be equally valued in the care planning process along with the expertise of professionals and practitioners.

What does this look like in practice?

- In the planning process, people are encouraged to pursue resources and planning activities within the community at large.

- Practitioners do not default to the "one-stop-shop" model of additional services or activities within the mental health setting, but instead use the question: "If I wanted to do x, where would I go?" as a helpful prompt to avoid continuing to rely solely on segregated or service settings.
- Practitioners get to know the options in the community, or know those people who are good "community connectors," in order to help people receiving services research options within their community of choice.
- Options such as Supported Housing, Supported Employment, Supported Education, Supported Socialization, Supported Parenting, and Supported Participation in Faith Communities are readily available and accessed in the planning process, if this level of support is necessary and desired by the person.
- Criteria for discharge to an independent community life or a lower level of care are clearly defined and are worked toward actively in the context of the service plan.
- Natural supporters are invited and welcomed according to the person's preference, in both the preplanning and care planning meetings.
- Practitioners support the person receiving services in identifying and expanding natural supports, using exercises such as the *Circle of Support* (see Module 3 for more details) or other tools designed to assist people in looking at their natural connections.
- Natural supporters such as friends and family members are given specific roles and follow-up steps in the plan, when applicable.

Responsible risk taking and growth are valued as part of recovery

In PCCP, individuals are presumed competent and entitled to make their own decisions. Prior to imposing power or restrictions, practitioners try multiple ways of engaging the person in this process. They support the dignity of risk and sit with their own discomfort as the person tries new experiences that are necessary for growth and recovery, working with the person to outline the range of existing options and their potential consequences and benefits.

> *A*ll human beings need the opportunity and freedom to learn from their own mistakes. Therefore, in circumstances that do not pose serious and imminent risks to the person or to others, direct supporters accordingly afford individuals "the dignity of risk" and "the right to failure."
>
> —*Deegan* [29]

Note that PCCP does not override a practitioner's ethical and societal obligation to intervene on a person's or the community's behalf should someone pose a serious and imminent risk to self or others. In such cases, just as in the case of an automobile accident or traumatic brain injury, health care practitioners are sanctioned to intervene on the person's behalf without getting prior consent. In mental health care, as in most other branches of medicine, however, such cases are the extremes and the exceptions, not the norm.

What does this look like in practice?

- Practitioners support the person in trying out new experiences while assisting and encouraging thoughtful decision making.

- Rights, for example, to refuse psychiatric medication (except, of course, in limited circumstances), are respected and privileges not denied for the person being served.
- Practitioners work to find the balance between *neglect*, letting the person "do whatever they want," and control/coercion, unnecessarily restricting rights and freedoms.
- Practitioners continue to abide by statutory obligations in the circumstances of potential serious or imminent harm to self or others or in circumstances of grave disability.
- Practitioners maximize the use of consumer-directed advance crisis planning tools (e.g., psychiatric advance directives that are described in greater detail in Module 8) to support people in taking responsible risks and to create contingency plans for how practitioners are to intervene (in a manner that is maximally consistent with the person's stated preferences) in the event of a crisis.

Focus of care and planning is on personally valued life goals

The plan itself is not the goal, even if it is multifaceted, culturally relevant, and directed by the person or family. Rather, the plan is simply one pathway to a life complete with respect from others, meaningful opportunities and choices, personal responsibility, community/school presence and participation, and self-chosen supports.

—Jonikas and colleagues [3]

Currently, it is common for planning efforts to focus largely, or exclusively, on the reduction of symptoms through the provision of professional clinical care. While these interventions continue to be an important part of overall care planning, PCCP also focuses on the attainment of broad-based life goals that the person decides are important to him or her. Areas such as physical health, family and social relationships, employment, education, parenting, spirituality, housing, recreation, and community service and civic participation are explored unless they are designated by the person as being not of interest.

In addition, clinical interventions are tied directly to the attainment of goals in a way that is clear to the individual and combined with other flexible supports as necessary. Whether the person's goal is to advance in the workplace or to audition for the lead character in a theater production, he or she should receive treatment and supports that promote the achievement of these personal goals. A practitioner's expertise is used in support of what is important to the person. For example, a psychiatrist or nurse practitioner who is considering medications needs to understand the individual's goals and in what ways taking medications will either help or hinder the person's efforts to reach those goals. Rather than simply assuming that because the person is ill he or she will necessarily need to take medication, and therefore writing out a prescription, the prescriber engages the person in a process of shared decision-making (SDM) in which he or she will then be able to make informed decisions about his or her own care.

Prescribing medications in this fashion often goes well beyond simply writing out a prescription. Employment-related goals may call for modifications to medication schedules to promote maximum energy and cognitive functioning at certain times during the day. The care team may need to discuss with the person how symptoms and/or medication side effects impact work performance and to brainstorm personal management strategies. If desired by the individual, the team can also contribute critical expertise in offering consultation to the employer regarding workplace environment that will enhance the individual's performance and potential for success. This example reflects how PCCP stresses using medication to promote maximum functioning in the workplace as opposed to using medication solely for the purpose of symptom reduction. Combined with other flexible supports, each of these interventions can be an important component of the ongoing PCCP process.

What does this look like in practice?

- Goals focus, when it is the person's preference, on quality of life areas such as work, housing, friendships, and so on.
- Interventions are linked closely to goal attainment, creating a cohesive narrative of the plan as it serves to help a person get closer to making changes in his or her life.
- Progress is measured not only by monitoring clinical outcomes (e.g., rates of hospitalization) but also by outcomes deemed meaningful by persons in recovery.

Cultural preferences and values individualize care

> It made such a huge difference to have my pastor there with me at my planning meeting. He may not be my father, but he is the closest thing I've got. He knows me better than anyone else in the world and he had some great ideas for me.
>
> —Practice Guidelines for Recovery-Oriented Behavioral Health Care—Connecticut Department of Mental Health and Addiction Services [30]

There is great diversity across cultures regarding the perception of mental illness and recovery. Similarly, the level of participation of people in PCCP is influenced by the person's cultural worldview. For example, the way an individual interprets symptoms and understands the origins of mental illness is often deeply rooted in cultural beliefs.

In an effort to honor diversity and support broad-based recovery goals, the PCCP process aims to offer people a flexible array of supports, including a wide range of different approaches such as self-management, peer support, holistic medicine, and cultural healers. These types of nontraditional supports should be made available for people in the manner that best assists them in their recovery. It is particularly useful to note strategies that have been helpful to others with similar struggles. Information about medications and other treatments should be incorporated with information about self-help, peer support, exercise, nutrition, daily maintenance activities, spiritual practices and affiliations, supported community activities, homeopathic and naturopathic remedies, and more. In some cases, this may require much creativity on the part of the team.

> *C*ulture includes, but is not limited to, the shared values, norms, traditions, customs, art, history, folklore, religious and healing practices, and institutions of a racial, ethnic, religious, or social group that are generally transmitted to succeeding generations.
> Cultural competence is a set of congruent practices, skills, attitudes, policies, and structures which come together in a system, agency, or among professionals and enable that system, or those professionals, to work effectively in cross-cultural situations.
>
> —Cross and colleagues [31]

Finally, as noted above, individuals from some cultural backgrounds that are more collectivist in nature may be uncomfortable with the values of personal control, autonomy, self-determination, and independence on which PCCP was originally based. Instead, family- and peer-centered processes are often more central to goal setting and decision making in these cultures. In these cases, practitioners must modify the PCCP process in a way that incorporates a more collective decision-making approach when it is necessary or desired.

What does this look like in practice?

- Culture is included and considered in all aspects of the planning and implementation of the plan, particularly in the assessment phase (see Module 4 for specific questions related to culture).
- A person's preference for family involvement is respected and encouraged.
- Cultural preferences for deferring to family members or others in making decisions are supported as individual choices.
- Practitioners reach out to faith and/or indigenous healers to better understand an individual's experiences of distress and recovery and include these healers/supporters in planning meeting when so desired by the service user.
- The practitioner makes efforts to educate and be curious about all cultures, including those that seem on the surface to be similar to his or her own.
- Agencies arrange for interpreters to participate in planning meetings, and for written recovery plans to be translated into a person's preferred language.

Stages of Change are considered in Recovery Planning

In order to best respect people's right to self-determination and to best assist as a facilitator in the PCCP process, it is, at times, useful to assess and consider a person's "readiness" to change. Several models have been developed to conceptualize and specify stages of change readiness so as to enable practitioners to try to match interventions to where the person may be along this continuum at any given time. Originally developed by Prochaska and DiClemente [32] to help account for behavioral change within the context of addiction, this framework has since been applied to numerous other health conditions, including mental illness. A couple of examples of such approaches are included in Table 2.1, along with the associated stages and recommended foci of treatment.

In applying such models to mental health recovery, there are at least two important considerations that must be taken into account. First, recovery is known to be a nonlinear process and therefore cannot be fully captured by such linear models as those described latter. Second, these models pertain to behavioral change, which is driven largely by the person's own choices; but choice plays a more limited, or at least different, role in mental health recovery than it does in addiction recovery. To put it simply, one cannot choose to be or not to be psychotic, that is, to experience psychotic symptoms such as hearing voices or feeling threatened, in the same way that one can choose to drink or not to drink alcohol or ingest or not ingest cocaine or heroin. Though we stress the role of personal choice in mental health recovery, the kinds of choices with which we are concerned are different and do not necessarily involve the kind of behavioral change required in addiction recovery.

Where, then, do stages of change and the "readiness" concept fit in? It may be useful to consider these kinds of stages in relation to specific aspects of recovery that do involve

Table 2.1   Stages of Change and Treatment Focus

Prochaska and DiClemente	The Village	State of Ohio	Stage of Treatment	Treatment Focus
Pre-contemplation	High risk/ unidentified or unengaged	Dependent unaware	Engagement	Outreach; practical help; crisis intervention; and relationship building
Contemplation/ preparation	Poorly cop-ing/engaged/ not self-directed	Dependent aware	Persuasion	Psychoeducation; set goals; and build awareness
Action	Coping/ self-responsible	Independent aware	Active treatment	Counseling; skills training; self-help groups
Maintenance	Graduated or discharged	Interdependent aware	Relapse prevention	Prevention plan; skills training; expand recovery

Adapted from Ref. [33].

behavioral change while keeping in mind that the overall process of recovery is neither linear nor under the person's control (i.e., many factors impact on recovery, such as genetic traits and social environment). For instance, the degree to which a person accepts that the voices he or she is hearing are auditory hallucinations that are symptoms of a major mental illness will certainly influence his or her willingness to take psychiatric medications. That specific component of his or her recovery might be usefully plotted out according to the stages above, moving from precontemplation ("I know that it is the devil speaking to me"), through contemplation ("It would be strange for the devil to have singled me out for this torture, perhaps there is something to what the doctors are telling me"), to action ("I'll try the medicine to see if it helps with the voices") and maintenance ("I know that when I start to hear the devil again it's time to talk to my doctor about adjusting my dose"). Understanding a person's current behavior and motivation in this way can be particularly useful in offering services that he or she may be more agreeable to, for example, a person in an early stage of recovery might welcome the opportunity to talk with a peer specialist about his or her experiences with medications but feel misunderstood or pressured if expected to participate in a medication-self-administration skills group.

In making such an application, however, it is important for the practitioner to take into account several common mistakes that are routinely made in practice. For example, it is important not to confuse the process of deciding to try medication with the person's overall recovery, as many people enter into and pursue recovery without the benefits of medication. Medications most often do not provide a cure, and about 30% of people with a psychotic disorder experience no relief from medications [34]. Therefore it would be a mistake to insist that a person take medication as a precondition for other supported activities, such as getting a job or going back to school, as these activities often provide a motivation *for* taking medication as well as have the added benefit of decreasing some of the same symptoms that would be targeted by the medication.

Similarly, it would be a mistake to assume that because the person is in a "precontemplative" stage with respect to accepting that hallucinations are symptoms of an illness, he or she must be in the same stage with respect to other important components of his or her recovery. The fact that people are instead more often in different stages in relation to different choices makes this a much more complicated and dynamic picture. This fact helps to account, for example, for why many people (over 70%) express a desire to work regardless of the level of symptoms they experience. As a result, helping someone to get a job can be an important first step in developing the kind of trusting relationship that will be a necessary foundation for PCCP, as well as for the person eventually to consider the possibility of taking medication. The same is true of assisting people with meeting other basic needs, such as those for safe and affordable housing, income, clothing, and physical health care. Making access to any of these basic resources contingent on the person doing whatever the practitioner thinks he or she needs to do in order to recover (e.g., taking medication, attending clinic appointments) is not only inconsistent with recovery principles but is unethical and, in certain circumstances, illegal.

In summary, while application of a stages of change model might be useful in relation to matching specific behavioral goals or components of recovery with specific interventions, practitioners are cautioned against linear interpretations as this is not consistent with the overall recovery process. The primary indicator of "readiness" for any particular activity or change is the person's own perspective on what he or she is interested in and able to do at any given time, not the result of a practitioner's assessment of symptoms or functioning levels. Recovery is something for which everyone is always already "ready" should there be a supportive social environment, encouraging and trusted others, and a modicum of self-efficacy and confidence in one's own abilities to take control of one's life, including one's mental health condition. What this recovery will look like, however, is different for each person. While for some it may appear to be an incremental process of gradual change in a relatively linear direction, for others it can be stimulated or facilitated abruptly by unforeseen events that enable people to start out in entirely new directions that practitioners could never have imagined. Here, as in most of PCCP, it is important for practitioners to exercise humility.

What does this look like in practice?

- Practitioners assess stages of change in relation to specific goals and specific components of recovery.
- Practitioners "program for success" by keeping the stage of change in mind when crafting short-term objectives, for example, objectives for someone in the precontemplative stage of change might be more modest and learning/motivation-based as compared to objectives for someone in the action stage which tend to be more action/behavior-based.
- Practitioners consider stage of change in suggesting services an individual may be interested in attending.
- Individuals are not "screened-out" of recovery and rehabilitation programs or services based on an assessment that they are not "ready" for participation (e.g., not clinically stable or complying with treatment, etc.).

Table 2.2 summarizes select person-centered practices that reflect each of the broader key principles discussed. In addition, the reader is referred to the section of Continuous Quality Improvement in Module 7 for a review of a comprehensive self-assessment tool, the *Person-Centered Care Questionnaire* [35], which evaluates the quality of PCCP from both a process and a documentation perspective.

Table 2.2   Select Representative Practices in PCCP

Key Principle	Select Representative Practices
Self-determination and community inclusion are fundamental human rights for all people	• Individuals are not required to attain, or maintain, clinical stability or abstinence before being supported by the care planning team in pursuing such goals as employment, education, or housing. • People are encouraged to pursue their recovery in whatever "order" or nonlinear fashion they choose, with the least number of "hoops" to jump through, for example, people have direct access to recovery services (e.g., supported employment, supported education) rather than being subject to "gate-keeping" where referral is controlled solely by a clinical practitioner.
Active participation and empowerment is vital	• The person receiving services has reasonable control over the nature and logistics of the planning process (e.g., when it occurs, who is involved). • Persons in recovery are offered training and education to build their knowledge of, and ability to actively partner in, all aspects of the PCCP process.
Developing trusting, reciprocal, and collaborative relationships is key	• Practitioners hold and convey hope that the person's life can be improved, for example, people are encouraged to "think big" in their recovery vision and goals are not discounted or judged as "unrealistic." • Practitioners take an active interest in the person's everyday life, in a conversational rather than interrogational manner, and help to identify and explore ways that life can be improved.
Language matters and should reflect recovery values	• "Person first" and verbatim language is used throughout documentation. • Generic labels (e.g., "low-functioning") are avoided and replaced with an objective description of how symptoms impact a person's life.
All parties have full access to the same information	• Language used in the plan is understandable to all, and when there is jargon, terms are explained to all involved. • The person receiving services is ALWAYS offered a copy of the plan.

(continued overleaf)

Table 2.2   (*continued*)

Key Principle	Select Representative Practices
Plans capitalize on strengths and the value of lived experience	• All care planning is based on a multidomain, strength-based assessment in order to identify abilities and supports in the process. • The recovery plan actively incorporates the person's identified strengths into the goals, objectives, or interventions.
High expectations for recovery are the norm	• Recovery plans do not default to "stability" or maintenance goals and objectives, but instead focus on the attainment of a meaningful life in the community. • Goal statements are not discounted as "unrealistic" but are seen as a reflection of ambitious expectations for recovery and an opportunity to inspire hope (even if such goals may need to be broken down into much smaller, modest objectives).
Natural community activities and relationships are emphasized	• Practitioners use the question: "If I wanted to do x, where would I go?" as a helpful prompt to avoid the "one-stop-shop" and continued reliance on segregated services. • Natural supporters are invited and welcomed according to the person's preference, in both the preplanning and care planning meetings.
Responsible risk taking and growth are valued as part of recovery	• Rights, such as the right to refuse psychiatric medication (except in limited circumstances), are supported without penalties. • Practitioners maximize the use of consumer-directed advance crisis planning tools (e.g., psychiatric advance directives) to support people in taking responsible risks and to create contingency plans for how practitioners are to intervene (in a manner that is maximally consistent with the person's stated preferences) in the event of a crisis.
Focus of care and planning is on personally valued life goals	• Goals focus, when it is the person's preference, on quality of life areas such as work, housing, friendships, and so on. • Interventions are linked closely to goal attainment, creating a cohesive narrative of the plan as it serves to help a person get closer to making changes in his or her life.
Cultural preferences and values individualize care	• Cultural preferences, for example, for deferring to family members or others in making decisions, is supported as an individual choice.

Table 2.2   (*continued*)

Key Principle	Select Representative Practices
	• Practitioners reach out to faith and/or indigenous healers to better understand an individual's experiences of distress and recovery and include these healers/supporters in planning meeting when so desired by the service user.
Stages of change are considered in recovery planning	• Practitioners assess stages of change in relation to specific goals and specific components of recovery. • Practitioners consider stages of change in suggesting services an individual may be interested in attending.

Exercises

Exercise 1. Essential Self-Reflection: Are You REALLY Already "Doing" PCCP?

 In orders to move forward in the implementation of person-centered recovery planning, it is necessary, first, to carry out an honest self-reflection on both previous and current planning practices. In doing so, we hope you will both appreciate the strengths to build on and acknowledge the areas in need of improvement.

Essential Self-Reflection in Person-Centered Planning

- Is there always a planning meeting? If so, who is usually in the meeting?
- Are individuals routinely given advance notice of their planning meetings?
- Who decides who needs to be at the meeting?
- How is the meeting organized? Who is in charge in setting the agenda and conducting the meeting?
- How often do meetings occur and what prompts these?
- Outside of regular meetings (e.g., every 3 or 6 months), are planned meetings ever called to address significant achievements and opportunities for new goal setting or are they limited to addressing crises or emergencies?
- What does the resulting care plan look like? What sections are included?
- What are the most common goals and objectives on care plans?
- How different do your plans look from one person to the next?
- How much of the plan is devoted to diagnosis and pathology as compared to strengths and resources?
- What kind of language does the plan use?
- What are the most common interventions included in care plans?
- Are there roles and action steps identified for the individual and his or her natural supporters?
- How do you monitor progress toward achieving the identified goals?
- Is it a common practice to offer a copy of the plan to the person? If not, what are the usual reasons for not doing so?

Exercise 2. The Language of PCCP: Glass Half Empty, Glass Half Full

 What types of messages might be communicated by the language used in the left column of Table 2.3? Identify a more strength-based term or phrase for each word while keeping

Table 2.3 Deficit Versus Strength-Based Language

	Deficit-Based Language	Strength-Based Alternative
1	A schizophrenic, a borderline	
2	An addict/substance abuser	
3	Clinical case manager	
4	Frontline staff/in the trenches	
5	Suffering from	
6	Treatment team	
7	High functioning versus low functioning	
8	Unrealistic	
9	Resistant/noncompliant	
10	Weaknesses/problems	
11	Maintaining clinical stability	
12	Treatment works	
13	Enable	
14	Frequent flyer	
15	Manipulative	

in mind the principles of strength-based language. How common are these terms in your everyday conversations and writing? Are there other words or phrases that you would like to change? Why?

	Deficit-Based Language	Strength-Based Alternative
1	A schizophrenic, a borderline	A person diagnosed with schizophrenia who experiences the following …
2	An addict/substance abuser	A person diagnosed with an addiction who experiences the following …
3	Clinical Case Manager	Recovery Coach/Recovery Guide (*I'm not a case, and you're not my manager!*)
4	Frontline staff/in the trenches	Direct care/support staff providing compassionate care
5	Suffering from	Working to recover from; experiencing; living with
6	High-functioning versus Low Functioning	Person's symptoms interfere with their relationship (work habits, etc.) in the following way …
7	Acting out	Person disagrees with Recovery Team and prefers to use alternative coping strategies

	Deficit-Based Language	Strength-Based Alternative
8	Unrealistic	Person has high expectations for self and recovery; ambitious
9	Denial, unable to accept illness, lack of insight	Person disagrees with diagnosis; does not agree that he/she has a mental illness precontemplative stage of recovery
10	Resistant/noncompliant	Not open to … Chooses not to … Has own ideas …
11	Unmotivated	Person is not interested in what the system has to offer; interests and motivating incentives unclear; preferred options not available
12	Decompensation, relapse	Person is reexperiencing symptoms of illness/addiction; an opportunity to develop and/or apply coping skills and to draw meaning from managing an adverse event; Reoccurrence
13	Maintaining clinical stability	Promoting and sustaining recovery
14	Puts self/recovery at risk	Takes chances to grow and experience new things
15	Noncompliant with medications/treatment	Prefers alternative coping strategies (e.g., exercise, structures time, spends time with family) to reduce reliance on medication; has a crisis plan for when meds should be used; beginning to think for oneself
16	Minimize risk	Maximize growth
17	Treatment works	Person uses treatment to support his/her recovery
18	Discharged to aftercare	Connected to long-term recovery management
19	Enable	Empower the individual through empathy, emotional authenticity, and encouragement
20	Frequent flyer	Takes advantage of services and supports as necessary
21	Dangerous	Specify behavior
22	Manipulative	Resourceful; really trying to get help
23	Entitled	Aware of one's rights
24	Baseline	What a person looks like when he/she is doing well
25	Helpless	Unaware of capabilities
26	Hopeless	Unaware of opportunities
27	Grandiose	Has high hopes and expectations of self
28	User of the system	Resourceful; good self-advocate

Exercise 3. Where We Are ... Where We Need to Go

Exercise 2 asked you to reflect on how we use particular words, but most of the time, these words are not used in isolation. Read the following narrative and highlight the words and statements that reflect a more deficit-based, traditional approach.

Where we are ...

Patient is a 43 year old schizophrenic with a long history of multiple psychiatric hospital-izations. For the last 18 months, patient has been compliant with meds and treatment. As a result, she has been clinically stable and has stayed out of the hospital. However, patient has not showed for last 2 visits and the team suspects she is off her meds. The Mobile Crisis Team was dispatched to her home today after patient failed to report to Clozaril clinic for blood-work.

- What kinds of words or statements did you highlight and why?
- How is the "where we are" narrative similar to the way people write notes or present "cases" at your agency? How is it different?
- If you are the Mobile Crisis worker, what might you be expecting during the home visit?
- How might the use of these words or statements affect the way services are rendered?

Next, consider the sample rewritten narrative below:
Where we need to go ...

In the last 18 months, Sandra has worked with her doctor to find meds that are highly effec-tive for her and she has been an active participant in activities at the clinic and the social club. Sandra and her team all feel as though she has been doing very well, e.g., returning to work, spending time with friends, and enjoying her new apartment. However, people have become concerned lately as she has been missed at several activities, including a blood work appoint-ment at today's clozaril clinic. The Mobile Outreach Team did a home visit to see if there was any way the clinic staff could assist her.

- What stands out, according to you, as the difference between the two narratives?
- How might the differences in language between the two narratives affect the way services are rendered?
- What other ideas do you have for how the narrative can be restoried?

Take home message:

Language counts! Person-centered language can exert a powerful influence on service delivery. Use of strengths-based, person-centered language communicates respect and the practitioner's belief in the person's capacity for recovery. This can become a self-fulfilling prophecy!

Exercise 4. Beware the Trap of the One-Stop-Shop

On a large piece of paper, list ALL the interventions, services, and supports that treatment/service systems provide. Think broadly and note EVERYTHING service recipients can access in mental health systems. Think about services/activities provided/sponsored by case managers, clinical/medical professionals, rehabilitation partners, family services, club-houses, drop-in centers, housing programs, and so on. Anything and everything available to people should be offered.

Now, consider the following questions:

- If a person did *not* have a mental health issue, where will he or she access these various activities in the community?
- Where do YOU, as a community member, access these things?
- Are individuals you support encouraged to make use of these same natural community and personal resources? If not, why?
- How do you encourage the creative use of natural resources in addition to all you offer within your service system?
- To what extent have you, or has your agency, developed partnerships/connections to community-based organizations, including those that are not mental health related?
- How might you go about establishing more of these types of connections and "tapping into" these community resources?

Take home message:

- Stigma/discrimination are NOT a reason to deny people access to, or to "protect" people from, the pitfalls (or potential joys) of community life.

Ask yourself: Am I about to recommend or create, in an artificial or segregated setting, something that can already be found naturally in the community?

Learning Assessment

Module 2: Key Principles and Practices of PCCP		
Statement	True	False
1. People receiving psychiatric treatment are unlikely to be able to decide their own recovery goals.		
2. Person-centered planning emphasizes connecting individuals with natural supporters and community activities.		
3. Practitioners are in the best position to develop goals and plans for individuals owing to their professional expertise and background.		
4. Only individuals who are clinically stable should be involved in making decisions about their care.		
5. It is harmful to have high expectations for individuals with mental illnesses.		
See the Answer key at the end of the chapter for the correct answers. **Number Correct**		
0 to 2: Don't be discouraged. Learning is an ongoing process! You can review the Module for greater knowledge. 3 to 4: You have a solid foundation. Use this Module to enhance your skills. 5: You are ahead of the game! Use this Module to teach others and strive for excellence!		

References

1. Tondora J, Pocklington S, Gregory GA *et al.* (2005) *Implementation of person-centered care and planning: How philosophy can inform practice.* Substance Abuse and Mental Health Services Administration, Rockville, MD.
2. O'Brien J. (2002). Numbers and faces: the ethics of person-centered planning. In Holburn S, Vietze PM (eds.), *Person-centered planning: Research, practice, and future directions* (pp. 399–414). Paul H. Brookes Publishing Co., Baltimore.
3. Jonikas J, Cook J, Fudge N *et al.* (2005) Charting a meaningful life: Planning ownership in person/family-centered planning. Paper presented at SAMHSA's National Consensus Initiative on Person/Family Center Planning Meeting on December, 8th 2005, Washington, D.C.
4. U.S. Supreme Court. (1891) Union Pacific Railway Co. v. Botsford, 141 U.S. 250 (1891) Union Pacific Railway Company v. Botsford No. 1375 Submitted January 6, 1891, Decided May 25, 1891, 141 U.S. 250.
5. Marrone J, Hoff D, Helm DT. (1997) Person-centered planning for the millennium: We're old enough to remember when PCP was just a drug. *Journal of Vocational Rehabilitation* **8**, 285–297.

6. SAMHSA. (2005) *Shared Decision Making in Mental Health Care*. Substance Abuse and Mental Health Services Administration, Rockville, MD.

7. Deegan PE. (2007) The lived experience of using psychiatric medication in the recovery process and a shared decision-making program to support it. *Psychiatric Rehabilitation Journal* **31**, 62–69.

8. Anthony W. (2003) Studying evidence-based processes, not practices. *Psychiatric Services* **54**, 7.

9. Davidson L, Strauss JS. (1992) Sense of self in recovery from severe mental illness. *British Journal of Medical Psychology* **65**, 131–145.

10. Connecticut Department of Mental Health and Addiction Services. (2008) *Practice Guidelines for Recovery-Oriented Care for Mental Health and Substance Use Conditions*. Connecticut Department of Mental Health and Addiction Services, Hartford, CT.

11. Deegan PE. (1992) The Independent Living Movement and people with psychiatric disabilities: taking control back over our own lives. *Psychosocial Rehabilitation Journal* **15**, 3–19.

12. Anthony W. (2004) Bridging the gap between values and practice. *Psychiatric Rehabilitation Journal* **28**, 105–106.

13. Davidson L, Stayner D, Haglund KE. (2008). Phenomenological perspectives on the social functioning of people with schizophrenia. In Mueser KT & Tarrier N (eds.) *Handbook of Social Functioning in Schizophrenia*. Allyn & Bacon Publishers, Needham Heights, MA, 97-120.

14. Deegan, PE. (1993). Recovering our sense of value after being labeled mentally ill. *Journal of Psychosocial Nursing and Mental Health Services* **31**, 7–11.

15. Deegan PE. (1994) A letter to my friend who is giving up. *The Journal of the California Alliance for the Mentally Ill*, **5**, 18–20.

16. Osher D, Keenan S. (2001) From professional bureaucracy to partner with families. *Reaching Today's Youth* **5**, 9–15.

17. Osher TW, Osher D. (2002) The paradigm shift to true collaboration with families. *Journal of Child and Family Studies* **11**, 47–60.

18. Winnicott DW. (1986) *Home is Where We Start From. Essays by a Psychoanalyst*. W. W. Norton, New York/London.

19. Sen A. (1999) *Development as Freedom*. Anchor Books, New York.

20. Copeland ME. (1997) *Wellness Recovery Action Plan*. Peach Press, Dummerson, VT.

21. Nerney T. (2005) Quality issues in consumer/family direction. Downloaded from www.mentalhealth.samhsa.gov/publications/allpubs/NMH05-0194/default.asp [July 13, 2005].

22. Nelson G, Ochocka J, Griffin K *et al.* (1998) Nothing about me, without me: Participatory action research with self-help/mutual aid organizations for psychiatric consumer/survivors. *American Journal of Community Psychology* **26**, 881–912.

23. Carling P. (1995) *Return to Community: Building Support Systems for People with Psychiatric Disabilities*. Guilford Press, New York.

24. Goldman HH, Ganju V, Drake RE *et al.* (2001) Policy implications for implementing evidence-based practices. *Psychiatric Services* **52**, 1591–1597.

25. Rowe M, Kloos B, Chinman M *et al.* (2001) Homelessness, mental illness, and citizenship. *Social Policy & Administration* **35**, 14–31.

26. Stein C, Wemmerus V. (2001) Searching for a normal life: Personal accounts of adults with schizophrenia, their parents, and well-siblings. *American Journal of Community Psychology* **29**, 725–745.
27. Reidy D. (1992) Shattering illusions of difference. *Resources* **4**, 3–6.
28. Bond GR, Becker DR, Drake RE *et al.* (2001) Implementing supported employment as an evidence-based practice. *Psychiatric Services* **52**, 313–322.
29. Deegan PE. (1996) Recovery and the conspiracy of hope. The Sixth Annual Mental Health Services Conference of Australia and New Zealand. Brisbane, Australia.
30. Connecticut Department of Mental Health and Addiction Services. (2006) *Practice Guidelines for Recovery-Oriented Behavioral Health Care*. Connecticut Department of Mental Health and Addiction Services, Hartford, CT.
31. Cross T, Bazron B, Dennis K *et al.* (1989) *Towards a Culturally Competent System of Care*, Volume **I**. Georgetown University Child Development Center, CASSP Technical Assistance Center, Washington, DC.
32. Prochaska JO, DiClemente CC. (1984) *The Transtheoretical Approach: Crossing Traditional Boundaries of Therapy*. Dow Jones-Irwin, Homewood, IL.
33. Adams N, Grieder D. (2005). *Treatment Planning for Person-Centered Care: The Road to Mental Health and Addiction Recovery*. Elsevier Academic Press, San Diego, CA.
34. Buchanan R, Kreyenbuhl J, Kelley D *et al.* (2010) The 2009 schizophrenia PORT psychopharmacological treatment recommendations and summary statements. *Schizophrenia Bulletin* **36**, 71–93.
35. Tondora J, Miller R. (2010) *Person Centered Planning: Information for Family Members and Supporters*. Unpublished handout. Yale Program for Recovery and Community Health, New Haven, CT.

Answers to the Learning Assessment:

1. F
2. T
3. F
4. F
5. F

Module 3: Preparing for the journey: Understanding various types of recovery plans and orienting participants to the PCCP process

Goal

This module introduces the various types of support plans and their roles within mental health service delivery systems. It describes the difference between person-centered care plans developed *within* service systems and other types of self-directed recovery plans that individuals might develop *outside* the context of professional treatment. In addition, it stresses the importance of providing PCCP education and "preplanning" activities to the individual and his or her invitees so that all stakeholders will have the necessary confidence and skills to be an active participant in the PCCP process.

Learning Objectives

After completing this module, the learner will be able to:

- describe the purpose and function of different types of plans for recovery, such as WRAP plans versus service or treatment plans;
- provide, as necessary, basic orientation to the individual and his or her natural supporter invitees regarding the purpose and process of person-centered care planning (PCCP);
- describe at least two legal protections that persons in recovery should be aware of as they pursue community-based PCCP goals;
- describe the potential role and activities of Peers in supporting the PCCP process;
- support individuals in carrying out necessary preplanning activities such as building a Recovery Team;

Partnering for Recovery in Mental Health: A Practical Guide to Person-Centered Planning, First Edition.
Janis Tondora, Rebecca Miller, Mike Slade and Larry Davidson.
© 2014 John Wiley & Sons, Ltd. Published 2014 by John Wiley & Sons, Ltd.

Learning Assessment

A learning assessment is included at the end of the module. If you are already familiar with the various types of recovery plans and how to prepare participants for their involvement in PCCP, you can go to the end of this module to take the assessment to test your understanding.

What Are the Different Types of Plans?

Different types of plans can be useful in supporting a person's recovery. Some might be described as self-help plans that can be created alone or with the assistance of family, friends, and other natural supporters. These "recovery" plans are often created *outside* the context of formal professional services, and the individual may, or may not, choose to share the plan with his or her treatment providers. In contrast, other types of plans (such as the "person-centered care plans, PCCPs" which are the focus of this text) are created *within* the context of professional services through a formal collaboration with a person's mental health care providers. The purpose and function of these different types of plans may vary, and an individual may elect to have one, the other, or both! Despite their unique characteristics, recovery and PCCPs share the same vision of helping an individual to move toward achieving his or her personally valued goals and aspirations.

WRAP and other recovery plans

A Wellness Recovery Action Plan™ (WRAP), developed by Mary Ellen Copeland, is one type of a self-directed recovery plan for identifying simple, safe, and effective wellness tools and strategies [1]. A WRAP can help a person to achieve whatever they want out of life, particularly if they want help managing their mental health issues and recovery. A WRAP can be created completely on one's own, but it may also be developed with the support of a peer-run educational program (see the list for further details regarding the role of a "peer support specialist, PSS") that aims to help people to S-H-A-P-E their lives through five principles of physical and emotional wellness:

Support
Hope
Advocacy
Personal Responsibility
Education

WRAP was developed through extensive data gathered from consumers of mental health services about the different approaches they had found to help them feel better and stay well. On the basis of that data, several people came together to create a simple system for recovery that has proven to be useful and effective for a wide range of people around the world [1]. For more information and resources regarding the WRAP, visit www.mentalhealthrecovery.com/.

In addition to WRAP, many systems of recovery planning have been created to help people create individualized wellness tools, which support them in accomplishing what they most want out of life. Some examples include:

- Pathways to Recovery: A Strengths Recovery Self-Help Workbook [2]
- This Is Your Life: Creating Your Self-Directed Life Plan [3]
- My Plan for Living Successfully [4]
- Personal Medicine [5]

WRAP and recovery plans are important self-help tools that people can create completely alone or with the help of family, friends, and other supportive individuals. What these plans have in common is that they prompt people to create their own personal vision of recovery and enable them to select the methods that they believe will work best for them as they pursue that vision. For many individuals, their recovery journey may include a path through the mental health treatment system. This brings with it the need for a different type of plan, that is, the required service or treatment plan.

Service or treatment plans

Service or treatment plans are documents that mental health professionals develop *within* the context of professional services in order to inform treatment and to meet system and regulatory obligations. These plans can help guide an individual's recovery by identifying valued life goals and the services and supports needed to attain those goals. Not only do these plans have clinical utility, but also are often used to meet the system requirements and standards of care. Most medical insurances, for example, reimburse providers and organizations only when there is clear documentation that their services or prescribed treatments are "medically necessary" (see Module 6 for more details regarding this concept) to help an individual to overcome identified problems associated with a mental health or addictive disorder. Treatment plans are also used to support utilization management, to authorize services, and to allocate limited resources.

Like any other complex system, these "requirements" of mental health service funders may be unintentionally counterproductive to the very service system they were originally intended to support. The service or treatment plans are often viewed as paperwork exercises required merely to fulfill regulatory demands but are otherwise of limited value to the consumer or provider. Practitioners openly express the frustration that treatment plans, as currently crafted, are not a meaningful part of the therapeutic work and partnership. In fact, many report that treatment planning actually interferes with their work and partnership given the heavy burden of documentation requirements they operate under (i.e., *We feel like we are treating the chart and not the person!*) and given the restricted and often negative content that currently dominates most plans (i.e., *People don't get excited about plans that only talk about med compliance and symptom reduction*).

In PCCP, however, an alternative vision is proposed where co-created treatment plans become a meaningful tool, for both the provider and the consumer, in shaping the person's unique recovery journey. PCCPs are fully informed by any personal action or recovery plan (such as a WRAP if the individual has elected to share this with his or her team) given the recovery-based principle of respect for both professional and lived experience. While a self-directed WRAP may *only include* personal wellness strategies (e.g., meditating, engaging in preferred hobbies, exercising), the PCCP, as discussed within this text, must *include* professionally delivered clinical and rehabilitative interventions as the PCCP is the "master document" that is meant to reflect a person's receipt of services within the mental health system. Table 3.1 outlines the key differences between a personal WRAP and a formal PCCP.

Table 3.1   WRAP Versus Person-Centered Care Plans

WRAP Plan	PCC Plan
A WRAP may be completed independent of the mental health system.	A PCC plan is completed within formal mental health services.
A WRAP dominant function is to support an individual's daily wellness and recovery.	A PCC plan serves an individual's recovery as well as multiple administrative and fiscal functions (e.g., the PCCP supports billing/payment for professional services rendered).
A WRAP belongs to the person in recovery. A person may, or may not, decide to share it with you as their clinician or provider. Information in a WRAP may be helpful in informing a treatment plan. People can be invited, but should not be required, to share their WRAP.	A PCC plan belongs to the team of people who have worked together to create it, that is, professionals, a service user, and his/her natural supporters. Professional members of the team automatically have access to the PCC plan as it is the formal document used to organize the delivery of mental health services and supports.
A WRAP identifies all the simple, safe, and effective things a person in recovery does to maintain their daily wellness. It also includes identifying things that may signal a crisis and how a person prefers such crisis situations to be handled, that is, who to involve, what services to offer, and so on.	A PCC plan identifies long-term goal(s) that might take months or even years to get to. It then identifies the short-term objective that will bring a person closer to his or her goal over the next 3 or 6 months. It may or may not include a crisis plan or any of daily wellness strategies that a person uses in his/her recovery.
A WRAP can be revised anytime, and the person in recovery decides when and how to use it.	A PCC plan can also be revised at any time. However, PCCPs are generally updated according to a standard schedule (e.g., every 3 months), which is determined by local and/or State regulations.
A WRAP focuses primarily on what the person in recovery will do to keep him- or herself well. While that may include the use of mental health services, the plan focuses on the individual's personal steps toward wellness.	A PCC plan must include the range of clinical and rehabilitative interventions that are provided to the person in recovery. Quality PCCPs also document self-directed action steps and contributions from natural supporters.

What is the Role of the Person in Recovery in PCCP and What Type of Orientation/Preparation is Helpful?

When developing a PCCP, as when developing a travel itinerary, sufficient attention has to be paid in advance to the planning process so that all those involved will know what to expect and how best to contribute as a member of the team. This advance education and "planning for the plan" increases the probability of long-term success and helps us evaluate whether or not we are satisfied with both the PCCP process and its hoped-for results.

A Cautionary Note Regarding Cultural Preferences and Person-Centered Care Planning

We offer an important cautionary note regarding the need to be attentive to cultural factors that may enter into the dialogue when providing education and preplanning support to individuals involved in PCCP. For those people from cultures or backgrounds where there is a more collectivist orientation, such as in many Latin, Native American, and African cultures, there may be questions and concerns about the individualistic nature of the planning process. These issues should be addressed right away, with the clear message that PCCP is meant to respect personal and cultural preferences for decision making, including when the preference is to defer to family members, elders, professional health care providers, or others. To insist that the individual assume primary responsibility for the process when he or she is not comfortable with that role is to ignore the very preferences the PCCP process is meant to elicit. When a person desires a more collective process, it should be honored in the spirit of tailoring care to his or her own cultural background, values, and priorities. Insisting otherwise can cause a rupture in the relationship and precipitate disengagement in services. Therefore, attending to this issue early and directly is essential.

PCCP is most effective when the individual and his or her natural supporters (e.g., family members, friends, spiritual guides) both understand and actively participate in all steps of plan development and implementation. Some individuals may naturally take the reins and engage in this process. Others may find person-centered planning to be a new or even uncomfortable experience. It is important for providers not to misinterpret this fear or discomfort as apathy, passivity, or a lack of motivation to engage in person-centered planning. An apparent reluctance to participate may, in fact, be due to the learned helplessness that stems from years of having other people take control and assume decision-making authority over one's life. Just as the process of sharing power and responsibility in treatment planning is a sometimes disconcerting shift in roles among mental health practitioners, many persons with psychiatric disabilities may truly want to exert greater control but feel unprepared to do so. Depending on the degree this contributes to the person's discomfort with "taking the wheel" in the recovery planning process, he/she might benefit from some "driver's education" regarding PCCP and how to be a partner within it. A toolkit for this purpose,

"Getting into the Driver's Seat: Preparing for Your Person Centered Plan" [6],[1] has been developed by the authors and used in multiple states to enhance the active involvement of persons in recovery in the PCP process.

This toolkit can be used to provide support and education so that persons in recovery are prepared to participate as much as possible as equal partners in the planning process. Many systems use sections of the toolkit during the intake procedures to orient individuals as to what to expect in treatment planning. In addition, it will be helpful to revisit the material closer to the time of an actual recovery planning meeting, as often people may be distressed or overwhelmed at their initial visit to a clinic or program. The toolkit can be reviewed individually or in the context of a facilitated PCCP preplanning group depending on the preferences of the person served. Finally, the toolkit contains multiple fillable worksheets, practice exercises, and educational handouts that all reinforce the importance of active participation in PCCP and build knowledge and competency in this area. Figure 3.1 provides a sample of one such handout designed as a simple take-home tool for persons in recovery.

Supporting the person to understand his or her rights

Person-centered planning is based on the fundamental premise that self-direction is, first and foremost, a human rights issue. Community inclusion, the right to exercise choice in where to live, who to love, how to worship, and what job to pursue are not choices that should be offered to someone only after they have achieved recovery (as determined by professional standards). These rights and freedoms are not contingent upon whether an individual is complying with treatment, finishing the day program, or proving abstinence or med compliance. They are inalienable human rights and must be valued as such throughout all phases of service design and delivery—including during the process of PCCP.

Service providers and administrators must themselves understand certain rights and freedoms individuals are entitled to so that they can, in turn, work to build this same knowledge among people in recovery. This knowledge is essential if persons in recovery are to engage in, and derive maximum benefit from, a PCCP. While there are a myriad of laws that protect the rights of persons living with mental illnesses, the following are particularly salient as they relate to the core purpose of PCCP, that is, the pursuit of recovery and a meaningful life in the community for all individuals.

> *P*eople in recovery have long been speaking out against assumptions that "to be mentally ill means to have lost the capacity for sound reasoning" or the capacity to take responsibility for their treatment and other major life decisions.
>
> —Deegan [7]

- **The right to self-direction** (1991 Consumer Self-Determination Act). This Act requires all Medicaid-funded facilities to offer opportunities to complete Advance Directives to all patients. What were initially conceptualized as documents primarily used to articulate in advance personal choices around death and dying have been expanded in most state statutes to include any treatment decisions during periods of incompetency as might be

---

[1] Available online at www.yale.edu/prch/personcentered.html.

Getting in the driver's seat of your treatment and recovery

Within your mental health care, a person-centered care plan, sometimes called a treatment plan or service plan, is the document that you create with your team to help plan how you want to move forward towards your personal goals.

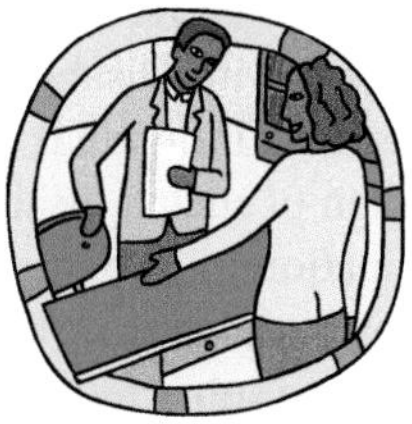

A person-centered care plan is used:
- to help decide on goals that are important to you in your recovery and well-being.
- to help decide on the things that you personally need to do to make progress toward these goals.
- to help decide on the types of services and supports your team can offer to help you achieve these goals.
- by your mental health team so they can document, and get payment for, the services and supports they provide to you.

A person-centered care planning meeting is a meeting:
- where you work in partnership with others to create your plan.
- that happens on a regular basis – usually every 3-6 months (although the plan can be updated as needed).
- where you have a right to invite anyone you would like to have involved. This can include professional staff (e.g., such as doctors, nurses, or therapists) as well as friends or family members.

For YOUR role in this meeting, it may be useful for you to:
- think about your priorities and goals ahead of time.
- think about your own responsibilities in working towards your goals.
- ask for the types of support that would be most helpful to you.
- bring up anything you think is important to you and what you want out of your life.
- discuss ways to pursue your goals, both treatment goals and also your goals and dreams for employment, education, social activities, and your living space.
- SPEAK UP and share your ideas and needs with your team!

After this meeting:
- your provider will work to include the things you talked about in a written document. This document is both a summary of the meeting and an outline of upcoming action steps for you and your team members (both professional providers and friends/family who may be involved).
- you should review the written plan with your provider and make sure you understand it. Ask questions if you don't.
- you should sign the plan and ask for a copy for your records. Keep it in a safe place to protect your own confidentiality.
- WORK YOUR PLAN! Follow through on your personal action steps and take charge of your life!

Figure 3.1   PCCP Orientation for People in Recovery

encountered during acute psychiatric crisis. Additional information regarding the use of these Psychiatric Advance Directives (PADs) as a tool of choice and self-direction is available from the National Resource Center on Psychiatric Advance Directives at: www.nrc-pad.org/.

The use of PADs in PCCP is strongly encouraged as they allow individuals to maintain certain degree of control over important decisions during clinical emergencies when control may need to be taken away temporarily for the safety of the individual and those around him/her. From the practitioner's perspective, PADs can be used as a more recovery-oriented risk management tool as they recognize a practitioner's obligation to step in and control a situation while at the same time giving the practitioner a meaningful tool to do so in a manner that is maximally respectful of the individual's choices and preferences.

- **The right to be free from discrimination** (The Americans with Disabilities Act, ADA, 1990). No qualified individual with a disability shall, by reason of such a disability, be excluded from participation in or be denied the benefits of the services, programs, or activities of any public entity or be subjected to discrimination by any such entity. The ADA explicitly prohibits discrimination against people with disabilities in employment, transportation, public accommodation, communications, and governmental activities. Knowledge of ADA rights and protections is essential as individuals seek to develop and enact their PCCP, which may involve deeply held desires to return to work, school, a faith community, a volunteer position, and so on.

> *This time, with a PAD, I did not receive any treatments that I did not want. They were very respectful. I really felt like the hospital took better care of me because I had my PAD. In fact, I think it's the best care that I've ever received.*
>
> —National Resource on Psychiatric Advance Directives
> www.nrc-pad.org/pad-stories

- **The right to live in the least restrictive environment** (Olmstead, 1999). Success in the community requires safe, affordable housing and appropriate support services, and the Olmstead decision has called on states to develop comprehensive plans to facilitate such community placements for institutionalized persons with disabilities. While Olmstead legislation is particularly relevant to PCCP as carried out in the context of hospital discharge planning, the underpinning value of supporting maximum independence and integration in the community alongside nondisabled persons should also inform the PCCP process as carried out in outpatient settings, for example, in developing a PCCP for an individual who would like to move out of a psychiatric rehabilitation group home into a supported apartment situation.
- **The right to live in the community** (The Fair Housing Acts of 1968 and 1988). Individuals have protection against housing discrimination based on disability and/or a number of other factors/characteristics. The Fair Housing Act of 1968 prohibits discrimination in the sale, rental, and financing of dwellings based on race, color, religion, sex, or national origin. The Act was amended in 1988 and expanded coverage to prohibit discrimination based on disability or on familial status (presence of child under age of 18 and pregnant women).
- **The right to education** (*Mills v Board of Education*, 1972) and the **Individuals with Disabilities Education Act (IDEA)**. The IDEA mandates that students with disabilities are educated in regular education settings to the maximum extent appropriate in light of their needs and prohibits their exclusion unless education there cannot be achieved satisfactorily even with appropriate supplementary aids and services. The IDEA protects children and transition-age youth with emotional disorders or psychiatric disabilities from the age of 3 to 21, while adults are protected from discrimination in educational settings under the ADA. For individuals who decide to pursue their education as a valued goal within their PCCP, knowledge of their legal rights and protections is needed both to ensure equal access to programs and to arrange possible classroom accommodations and supports after enrollment.

Involvement in PCCP often inspires people to resume, or pursue for the first time, valued goals and activities they previously may have felt to be unattainable. With this growth and opportunity comes the risk of possible exposure to stigma and discrimination. Collectively, these various laws provide protections against discrimination for persons with mental illness who identify the pursuit of employment, housing, education, and other community activities as high priority recovery goals. In providing orientation to the PCCP process, individuals must be made aware not only that such laws exist, but also about where to go for help in the event they believe their rights have been violated. For additional information on these, and other relevant pieces of legislation that protect the rights of individuals with psychiatric disabilities, see the Bazelon Center for Mental Health law at www.bazelon.org, the UPENN Collaborative on Community Integration at www.upennrrtc.org, and the National Disability Rights Network (NDRN) at www.ndrn.org/index.php. These organizations can provide information, referral, and advocacy services in the event a person has been the subject of discrimination or other unlawful treatment.

In summary, in order for persons in recovery to be full participants in PCCP, it may be necessary to offer education before, during, and after the process. People receiving services may never have experienced a person-centered approach before, and may need help understanding the expectations of their roles within it. Similarly, people may be unaware of the new opportunities that PCCP can bring and unaware of the range of laws that will protect and support them as they pursue these opportunities. No matter what one's experience with PCCP, nearly all programs, service settings, and individuals can benefit from certain preparatory activities that can be conducted prior to the planning meeting itself. Doing so will increase the likelihood that the plan will be a positive and productive experience for all involved.

Sample preplanning questions and activities that will prepare people to be as active and empowered as possible in their PCCP meeting might include encouraging the individual to:

- Review the current recovery plan to reflect on progress made since the last planning meeting and to determine if changes in goals and supports are desired.
- Share this plan with a trusted other to receive feedback and ideas.
- Decide if they would like to invite someone to support them in their planning meeting by considering the questions: Who can help you to get what you want? Who do you trust? (See *Circle of Support* activity below for more details).
- Ask individuals the persons they would like to attend and what times would be more convenient for them to be involved.
- Speak up if there is anyone they feel should not be in attendance at their planning meeting.
- Identify the most important priority areas in need of attention.
- Make note of the most important things they want to communicate in the meeting.
- Think how they will communicate during the meeting if they are happy or unhappy about what is being said or talked about.

Now that we have presented an overview of *what* type of information regarding PCCP would be most helpful, *who*, then, is in the best position to provide this essential education and preplanning support to persons in recovery? While this can be offered by any individual who is knowledgeable in the principles and practices of PCCP, it is particularly effective to call upon the mentoring skills of peer specialists who have prior experience with PCCP and who have used it as a successful tool in their own recovery.

What is the role of the peer in the PCCP process?

What is a Peer Support Specialist?

The national Peer-to-Peer Resource Center (see www.peersupport.org/) describes a PSS as **a person with a mental illness who has been trained to help her/his peers—other people with mental illnesses—to identify and achieve specific life goals**.

A PSS promotes self-determination, personal responsibility, and empowerment inherent in self-directed recovery, and assists people with mental illnesses in regaining control over their own lives and over their own recovery process. As someone who has experienced a mental illness himself or herself, the PSS role-models recovery and maintenance of ongoing wellness.

PSSs generally work for pay in a range of mental health settings. They may be employees of a mental health agency, a peer-run agency, or their services may be contractually purchased. Finally, PSSs may also be trained volunteers who wish to give back to others as a part of their own recovery process.

The peer-to-peer model is an exceptional example of the innovative ways in which we can help the system overcome its own barriers. Peer-support programs are not just empowerment programs. They are an expression … and an example … of the way the system is going to have to fundamentally change to foster healing relationships, and create an environment conducive for recovery.

Kathryn Power, Director, Center for Mental Health Services

PSSs can play a unique role in the PCCP process as teachers and coaches in either group or individual settings. Some agencies have hosted monthly educational PCCP potlucks while others have set aside peer specialists "office-hours" where people can sign up for 1:1 sessions to review PCCP materials and prepare for upcoming recovery planning meetings. While some service users prefer "behind the scenes" support in advance, others may prefer the peer specialist to accompany them to the actual planning meeting to provide additional support around communicating preferences and developing an action plan. Bellamy and colleagues [8] have developed an 8-session group curriculum for use by peer specialists to introduce key PCCP practices, outline expectations of the provider and the person receiving services, and help begin the process of exploration in setting goals and priorities. A group setting can also provide inspiration to individual participants, especially for those who feel stuck in identifying the next steps or hopes and dreams. Peer specialists often use the embedded resources of the *Driver's Seat Toolkit* in carrying out various types of individual or group-based PCCP education.

For example, drawing on the experiences of Canadian inclusion advocates and researchers, the Toolkit exercise, *Building Your Circle of Support*, can be helpful to complete in order to identify those individuals who may be invited to be a part of the recovery team and the

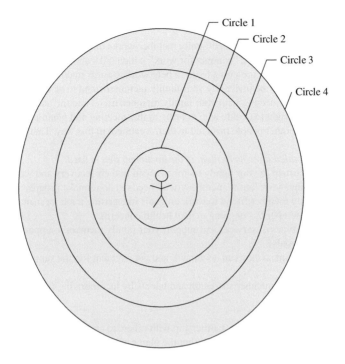

Circle 1

Circle 2

Circle 3

Circle 4

Figure 3.2 Building Your Circle of Support [9]

PCCP process. This tool, shown in Figure 3.2, provides a template of concentric circles to use as a visual representation of relational closeness with those in Circle 1 representing a sphere of intimacy (people dear to us with whom we share our deepest secrets and emotions) and those in Circle 4 representing a sphere of more distant affiliation or exchange (people we may know but are not close to). The idea is to identify in broad strokes those people who matter in someone's life, with the eventual goal of selecting those supporters who the person receiving services would like to involve in the PCCP process. The potential value of building a recovery team involving both informal (friends, family members, etc.) and formal supports (a psychiatrist, therapist, employment specialist, etc.) is discussed further in this module, and is consistent with the recovery-based practice of facilitating natural community connections and relationships as a source of healing whenever possible.

For some people receiving services, the Circles exercise can bring up many strong feelings, especially for those who are estranged from family and friends and who feel they do not have enough support in their lives at the current time. This can lead to an important conversation about one potential of PCCP: being a means of repairing, or building a new, recovery-promoting relationships. It is also an opportunity for the provider to be creative and think broadly with the person about who actually in his or her life may contribute to the plan. In the Circle of Support exercise, it is important to consider a wide variety of people and contacts, including some who may not typically be considered, like the counter clerk at the coffee shop, the mail carrier, and others, as it may be the counter clerk who arranges for a part-time job for the individual and the mail carrier who offers to knock on the individual's door each day to make sure they are on time!

Person Centered Planning: Information for Family Members and Supporters

As part of receiving treatment, your friend/family member works on a document called a *treatment plan* or *recovery plan*. This plan is a "contract for work" which talks about what your family member/friend and their treaters are going to do to help work towards making your friend/family member's life better. You may be invited by your family member/friend to be a part of the planning process, or even to attend a meeting with your family member/friend and the team. Your family member or friend has the right to decide who to bring to this meeting and planning process. Some people prefer to not have other people involved in their treatment in this way. That is also their right.

A treatment plan, also called a recovery plan, is the document that is used:
- To identify goals important to your family member/friend in their recovery and well-being.
- To help decide on things your family member/friend needs to do to make progress on these goals.
- To support your family member/friend to work on goals like getting a job, or managing money, even if your family member has ongoing mental health concerns.
- To help decide on the types of services and support your family member's support team can offer to help achieve these goals.
- By the mental health team so they can document, and get payment for, the supports they provide to your family member.
- To build upon your family member's strength and talents by incorporating them in his/her plan.

A "recovery planning" meeting is:
- Where your family member works in partnership with others to create the treatment plan.
- On a regular basis, often every 3–6 months (but the plan can be updated as needed).
- Where your friend/family member should feel comfortable and respected.
- Where your friend/family member gets education on personal wellness strategies and peer support.
- Where your friend/family member has the right to invite anyone they would like, including doctors or therapists as well as friends or family members.
- An opportunity for staff to learn about cultural factors (such as spiritual beliefs and cultural views) that are important to your friend/family member, and how to include those in the plan.

If your family member/friend desires, you can be a support in numerous ways. These might include.
- Helping your friend/family member think about priorities and goals ahead of time.
- Asking your friend/family member what kinds of support would be helpful for them.
- Offering support and assisting your family member in advocating for themselves.
- Respecting your friend/family member's wishes and rights.
- Following through on action steps on the plan, such as practical help with transportation.

What happens after this meeting?
- The clinician will work to include the things talked about in a written document.
- Your family member should be offered a copy of the plan.
- The treatment plan should be written so that your friend or family member can understand it, and words that are not understandable are explained.

© Tondora and Miller, 2010.

Figure 3.3   PCCP Orientation for Family Members and Other Natural Supporters

> *Family members and friends are often an important aspect of people's recovery. Person Centered Planning is one tool that the mental health system uses to assist your friend or family member in getting the support they need. This educational handout tells you information about Person Centered Care Planning that you should know:*

Once potential PCCP participants are identified, possibly through the completion of the Circles exercise, each person's respective role—whether they are a friend, family member, or other natural supporter—should be thought out with the person receiving services and made clear before the planning process begins.

What is the role of the natural supporter in PCCP and what type of orientation/preparation is helpful?

Orientation should also be provided to natural supporters who may wish to be involved in the PCCP process. Figure 3.3 provides a sample of an informational handout that can be used for this purpose. While a recovery-oriented system strives to tap into, and/or build, one's natural support network, it can bring up difficult tensions as involvement of friends and family must be at the discretion of the service user. If an individual prefers to keep their planning meetings more private, this decision must be respected and invitations to natural supporters should not be issued without the permission of the service user.

In such cases, awareness of the person's rights may be essential in supporting his or her desire for self-determination and privacy. In addition, when a person does desire, and consent to, the active participation of family members or friends, these natural supporters need advance education regarding their role and what is expected of them in the meeting. For example, it is essential that all understand that the PCCP meeting is not an opportunity for the team to "gang up" on an individual and convince him/her to follow a certain path that others believe is in his or her best interest. While everyone involved is given an opportunity to share his/her perspective and ideas, the team needs to guard against this group dynamic so that the person receiving services does not experience undue pressure to concede to the will of the majority. The likelihood of this type of conflict arising can be decreased by providing natural support participants with advance orientation regarding the ground rules for respectful and inclusive PCCP meetings.

Despite a provider's best efforts to offer this advance orientation, further redirection may be necessary during the course of the actual meeting if the family member or natural supporter begins to challenge or disagree with the person receiving services in a counterproductive manner (see Module 5 for more details). As a means of preparing for such situations, it is helpful for the provider and/or PSS to check in with the person in recovery ahead of time to find out how he or she would like to see the meeting managed, what would signal that things are going badly, and how the PCCP facilitator can step in and refocus the conversation if needed.

Exercises

Exercise 1. Consider the following questions:

1. Think about your agency's intake and orientation procedures. What types of information have they given about their rights and responsibilities in recovery planning? What are the relative strengths and weaknesses of your orientation materials and process?

2. Do individuals have access to supports in order to prepare for their person-centered planning meeting? If not, how might you use the information in this module to build these supports?
3. To what extent are you familiar with the types of rights and legal protections described earlier? Were you aware that they applied to individuals with psychiatric disabilities?
4. To what extent do you think the people you serve are familiar with the types of rights and protections described?
5. Can you describe examples where these rights and protections have been violated—either inside the mental health system or in individuals' community experiences?
6. How did you (or your agency) respond to that situation? How might you respond now?
7. What types of activities (at the agency level or at the level of the individual service provider or service user) can build capacity to recognize, and respond to, instances of rights violations?

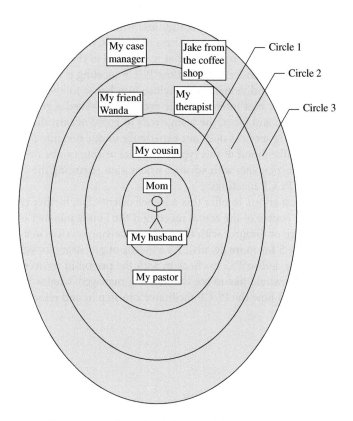

Figure 3.4   Sample of Circle of Support Exercise

Circle 1. People you love, people who love you, people you would not want to live without
Circle 2. Close friends or relatives, people you count on, people you trust most
Circle 3. People you know from clubs, hobbies, work, etc.
Circle 4. People who are meaningful to you but with whom you are not that close
Start at the outside and work your way in.
(People can be in more than one circle at a time.)

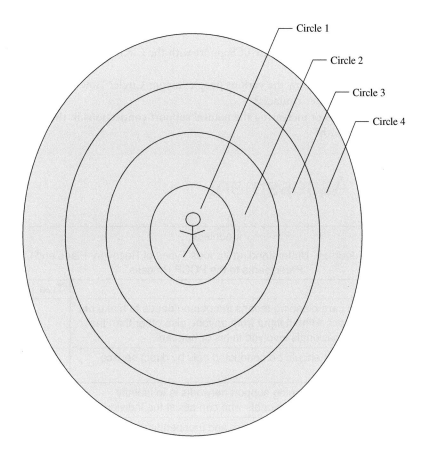

Figure 3.5 Template for Circle of Support Exercise

Exercise 2. Circle of Support Exercise

The Circle of Support exercise can be a useful tool to help people receiving services identify who is important in their life and who they would like to be a part of their support team in PCCP. Each expanding concentric circle indicates degree of closeness. See Figure 3.4 for a sample circle already filled out, with some possible responses by a person in recovery. Take a look at this sample.

Following the completed example, Figure 3.5 is a blank form for you to try filling out.

Some guidelines that might help in completing this tool are as follows:

- What was your experience of filling out the Circle of Support? What did you find easy? Difficult?
- Now, complete a second circle for an individual with whom you work. Pick someone you know well and complete the circle based on your knowledge of the individual's network. Start at the outside and work your way in.
  - Compare and contrast your Circle of Support with the Circle of the individual whom you support.
  - How did you come to know the various people in your Circle? How did the service user come to know his or her contacts?
  - What are some ways of increasing the natural support connections in the lives of the people you work with?

Learning Assessment

Module 3:		
Preparing for the Journey: Understanding Various Types of Recovery Plans and Orienting Participants to the PCCP Process		
Statement	True	False
1. Person-centered care planning means the person needs to make his or her own decisions without input from anyone else other than the mental health professionals involved in his or her care.		
2. Preplanning activities should be conducted only by direct service providers.		
3. The primary goal of developing support networks is to identify additional paid service professionals who can assist the individual.		
4. Personal autonomy, self-determination, and independence may be values inconsistent with an individual's cultural worldview.		
5. Orientation and education regarding PCCP is not necessary for any individual receiving services.		
See the Answer Key at the end of the chapter for the correct answers. **Number Correct**		
0 to 2: You have a lot to learn, but we hope you find this guide useful in the process! 3 to 4: You have a solid foundation. Use this guide to enhance your skills and the supports you offer. 5: You are ahead of the game! Use this guide to teach others and strive for excellence.		

References

1. Copeland ME. (1997) *Wellness Recovery Action Plan*. Peach Press, Dummerson, VT.

2. Ridgway P, McDiarmid D, Davidson L *et al.* (2002) *Pathways to Recovery: A Strengths Self-Help Workbook.* University of Kansas, School of Social Welfare, Office of Mental Health Research and Training, Lawrence, KS.
3. Jonikas J, Cook J. (2004) *This is your Life! Creating your Self-Directed Plan.* UIC NRTC Self-Determination Series. University of Chicago, Chicago, IL.
4. Depression and Bipolar Support Alliance. (2006) *My guide to living successfully.* Downloaded from http://www.dbsalliance.org
5. Deegan PE. (2005) The importance of personal medicine: a qualitative study of resilience in people with psychiatric disabilities. *Scandinavian Journal of Public Health* **33**, 29–35. *Olmstead v. L.C.*, 527 U.S. 581 (1999).
6. Tondora J, Miller R., Guy K *et al.* (2008) *Getting in the Driver's Seat: Preparing for your Person-Centered Plan.* Unpublished workbook. Yale Program for Recovery and Community Health, New Haven, CT.
7. Deegan PE. (1992) The independent living movement and people with psychiatric disabilities: taking control back over our own lives. *Psychosocial Rehabilitation Journal* **15**, 3–19.
8. Guy K, and Bellamy CD (2009). *Guidebook on Facilitating a Person-Centered Planning Group: Promoting Recovery-Oriented Dialogues Among People in Recovery.* Yale Program for Recovery and Community Health, Yale University, New Haven.
9. Falvey MA, Forest M, Pearpoint J and Rosenberg RL (1997). *All my life's a circle: Using the tools: Circles, MAPS & PATHS.* Toronto, Canada: Inclusion Press.

Answers to the Learning Assessment:

1. F
2. F
3. F
4. T
5. F

Module 4: Strength-based assessment, integrated understanding, and setting priorities

Goal

This module offers information regarding the completion of a culturally appropriate, strength-based assessment that can inform the development of a person-centered recovery plan.

Learning Objectives

After completing this module, you will be able to:

- name at least three principles of strengths-based assessment;
- identify the range of questions included in a culturally competent, strength-based assessment;
- understand the difference between assessment data and the integrated understanding;
- support individuals in carrying out necessary preplanning activities such as identifying and prioritizing goals;
- explain the concept of important *to* versus important *for* and how this applies to person-centered care planning.

Learning Assessment

A learning assessment is included at the end of the module. If you are already familiar with the topics presented, you can go to the end of this module to take the assessment to test your understanding.

Partnering for Recovery in Mental Health: A Practical Guide to Person-Centered Planning, First Edition.
Janis Tondora, Rebecca Miller, Mike Slade and Larry Davidson.
© 2014 John Wiley & Sons, Ltd. Published 2014 by John Wiley & Sons, Ltd.

Building a Person-Centered Plan

As illustrated in Figure 4.1, the creation of a person-centered plan can be organized into several logical steps that follow in order and include:

- Conducting a strengths-based assessment;
- Formulating an integrated understanding of the individual;
- Prioritizing the areas to be addressed;
- Setting recovery goals and a vision for the future;
- Identifying barriers as well as strengths to draw on;
- Creating short-term objectives that help to overcome barriers;
- Describing interventions or activities reflecting a range of evidence-based and emerging practices;
- Evaluating progress and outcomes (including evaluating discharge/transition criteria);
- Keeping a medical record that reflects all these.

After an individual's entry into care, the next step in the development of a person-centered care plan (PCCP) is the comprehensive *assessment*. The assessment provides the foundation for a plan, but it is not meant to be an interrogation. In PCCP, as mentioned in Module 3, the focus is on a *strength-based* assessment process and product. PCCP must begin where each individual is at the time, as "no matter how person-centered a practice is in theory, it ceases to be person-centered if it does not respect the individual's preferences as well as his or her existing capacities and resources" [1]. Discussion of strengths is a central focus of every assessment, care plan, and case summary. Assessments begin with the assumption that people are the experts on their own life experiences and that they have learned much in the process of living with and working through their struggles. Focusing solely on deficits in the absence of a thoughtful analysis of strengths disregards the most critical resources an individual has on which to build in his or her efforts to advance in his or her recovery. The strength-based planning in PCCP is based on the "Strengths Model" developed by Rapp [2].

Within a strength-based model, those providing support help the individual or family to identify the strengths they can draw on to set goals and plan activities. This emphasis on

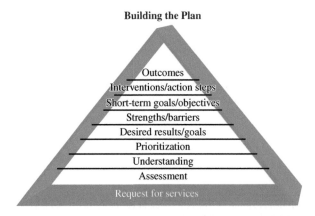

Figure 4.1   The Logic of Building a Plan (from Ref. [8]). Reproduced with permission from Elsevier Academic Press

personal and/or family "strengths," instead of a focus on deficits or problems, is sometimes a difficult shift for providers, natural supporters, and people in recovery alike to make. It is not uncommon, for example, for individuals to have difficulty identifying their "strengths" as this has not historically been the focus of mental health services and assessments. As a result, individuals may have lost sight of their gifts and talents through years of struggle (both with the illness and with the discrimination associated with it). In these cases, simply asking the question "What are your strengths?" may not be enough to elicit information regarding resources and capabilities that can be built on in the planning process. The following section describes the guiding principles and sample questions for engaging in a strength-based assessment process.

Guiding Principles of Strength-Based Assessment

Here are 10 guiding principles for a strength-based assessment process.

Collaborate

The strength-based assessment is conducted as a collaborative process, and all assessments in the written form, or through verbal discussion, are shared with the individual.

Ask asset-based questions

Initial assessments recognize the power of simple, yet powerful, questions such as "What happened?" "What do you think would be helpful?" "What are your goals in life?" and "What would make things better for you?" Self-assessment tools rating the level of satisfaction in various life areas can be useful to identify diverse goal areas for which supports can then be designed.

Reframe "negatives" as potentially transferable skills

Providers attempt to reframe perceived deficits within a strength-based framework, as this will allow the individual to identify less with the limitations of his/her disorder. For example, identifying the resourcefulness required to survive in the midst of an addiction can reframe what had been perceived as shameful as a strength the person can now draw on in a positive manner while striving for recovery. Particularly for those who have experienced severe trauma, reframing experiences and even symptoms as adaptations and potentially transferable skills can be highly therapeutic in the recovery process.

Draw on social capital outside of the mental health system

While the strengths of the individual are a focus of the assessment process, thoughtful consideration is given also to the potential strengths and resources within the individual's family, natural support network, service system, and community at large. This is consistent with the view that recovery is not a solitary process but rather a journey toward interdependence within one's community of choice.

Explore diverse strengths

The diversity of strengths that can serve as resources for the person and his or her planning team is respected, and areas not traditionally considered "strengths," are fully explored, for example, the individual's most significant or most valued accomplishments, sources of joy and contentment, ways of relaxing and having fun, ways of calming down when upset, preferred living environment, educational achievements, personal heroes, most meaningful compliment ever received, and so on. Saleeby [3] recommends structuring the strength-based-interview according to the following dimensions:

Skills such as gardening, caring for children, speaking Spanish, and doing budgets.
Talents such as playing the bagpipes, cooking, painting, and sewing.
Personal virtues such as insight, patience, sense of humor, and self-discipline.
Interpersonal skills such as comforting others and mediating conflicts.
Interpersonal resources such as extended family and supportive neighbors.
Cultural knowledge such as healing rituals and stories of cultural perseverance.
Family stories and narratives such as migration and settlement, and redemption.
Overcoming adversity such as surviving past events, and maintaining hope and faith.
Occupational or parental roles such caring for others and planning events.
Spirituality and faith or a system of meaning to rely on and granting a purpose beyond
   oneself.

Assess needs and resources in multiple life spheres

Assessment explores the whole of people's lives while ensuring emphasis is given to the individual's expressed and pressing priorities. For example, people experiencing problems with mental illness or addiction often place less emphasis on symptom reduction and abstinence than on desired improvements in other areas of life such as work, financial security, safe housing, or relationships. For this reason, it is beneficial to explore in detail each individual's needs and resources in these areas.

Include personally identified strategies in the plan

Strength-based assessments ask people what has worked for them in the past and incorporate these ideas in the plan. People are more likely to use strategies that they have personally identified or developed rather than those that have been prescribed for them by others. These strategies may be solicited informally in conversation or may be captured in more structured daily wellness approaches such as Wellness Recovery Action Planning (WRAP), which is widely respected as a highly effective, person-directed recovery tool (see Module 3 for more details on WRAP).

Implement solution-focused approaches

Guidance for completing a strength-based assessment may be derived from certain inter-viewing strategies employed within the solution-focused approaches to treatment. For example, DeJong and Miller [4] recommend the following types of inquiry: exploring for exceptions (occasions when the problem could have occurred but did not); imagining a future when the problem has been solved and exploring, in detail, how life would then be different; assessing coping strategies, for example, asking how an individual is able to cope despite the presence of such problems; and using scaling questions (where the person rates his or her current experience of the problem) to elucidate what might be the subtle signs of progress.

Avoid simplistic cause and effect explanations

Cause and effect explanations are offered with caution, if at all, in strength-based assessment, as such thinking can lead to simplistic resolutions that fail to address a person's situation. In addition, simplistic solutions may inappropriately blame the individual for a problem, with blame being described as "the first cousin" of deficit-based models of practice [5]. For example, to conclude that an individual did not pay his or her rent as a direct consequence of his or her "noncompliance" with medications could lead to an intrusive intervention to exert control over the individual's finances. Strength-based assessments respect that problem situations are usually the result of complex, multidimensional influences and explore with the person in detail the various factors that led to his or her decisions and behavior (e.g., expressing displeasure with a negligent landlord).

Expand the assessment over time as needed

Strength-based assessments are developed through in-depth discussions with the individual as well as attempts to solicit collateral information regarding the strengths from the indi-vidual's family and other natural supports. Obtaining all the necessary information and a trusting relationship with the person requires time, and a strength-based assessment may need to be completed (or expanded on) after the initial contact as treatment and rehabilita-tion unfold. While each situation may vary, the assessment is written up as soon as possible in order to help guide the work and interventions of the PCCP team.

The Role of Culture in Assessment and Formulation

Just as it is important to consider how culture might impact an individual's preferred role in the PCCP process, it is equally critical to conduct all assessments in a culturally sensitive manner. Although often overlooked, the *DSM-IV-TR* [6] provides a simple, but useful, out-line of what should be included in considering cultural factors and how they influence both the assessment and the PCCP:

Cultural identity: *Cultural reference groups; language(s); cultural factors in development; involvement with culture of origin; and involvement with host culture.*

Cultural explanations of illness: *Idioms of distress; meaning and severity of symptoms in relation to cultural norms; perceived causes; and help-seeking experience and plans.*

Cultural factors related to psychosocial environment and levels of functioning: *Social stressors; social supports; and level of functioning and disability.*

Cultural elements of the provider-person relationship: *Provider's ethnocultural background; language; and knowledge of person's culture.*

For practitioners interested in exploring further the cultural factors and their impact on an individual's experience of care, the questions in Table 4.1 are offered as samples of a more culturally sensitive method of "Bio-Psycho-Social Assessment" [7]. These questions prompt the practitioner to explore culturally meaningful life areas, including the person's belief in God and participation in religious services; important relationships and supporters, including sexual relationships; experiences of emigration and discrimination; ethnic identity and participation in cultural celebrations; and language of preference. In addition, at the end of this module is a sample of a more comprehensive person-centered and culturally appropriate interview guide. These types of interviews can be used to stimulate the recovery goal identification that is essential in any quality PCCP process.

Table 4.1 Sample Questions for Culturally Appropriate Assessment

• What do you call your situation? What brings you here, to services, and how did you end up in this situation?
• Who do you include as family? Who do you trust?
• Have you ever been a member of a faith community?
• Are you a member of a faith community now? If so, would you like the Rabbi, Priest, Pastor, Imam, and such others involved in your support network?
• Are you now going, or have you ever gone, to an Indigenous healer for help with your problem? Would you like that person involved as part of your recovery support network?
• With whom do you have intimate relations and relationships?
• Have you ever experienced racism, police brutality, discrimination, and/or other forms of oppression?
• How do you identify yourself culturally/racially/ethnically?
• What do you know about your culture? What holidays do you observe? Are they related to your culture?
• Has your family always lived in this area?
• What messages did you receive about your culture while growing up?
• What messages did you receive about the cultures of others?

Importance of Understanding

Data collected during the assessment process is by itself *not sufficient* for recovery planning. Some sort of integrated summary, formulation, or understanding is also necessary. Developing this kind of understanding typically requires some degree of technical skill and experience (clinical judgment) and should always include some consideration of the role of culture and ethnicity as critical to achieving a full and accurate appreciation of the person served.

The integrated summary of assessment data is more than a retelling of the facts. The formulation helps move both the individual and the provider from thinking about *what* to considering *why*. In doing so, the integrated formulation can set the stage for prioritizing the needs and goals as well as suggesting solutions to the barriers and challenges that have led the individual to seek help. One common quality error in the integrated formulation is to limit the narrative to a mere summary or repetition of the data. Consider someone who routinely has not used his/her psychiatric medications effectively in the community, which has contributed to a revolving-door pattern of repeated hospitalizations. After this history has been detailed within the assessment, it is not uncommon to see this restated within the integrated summary; for example, "the patient is a 52-year-old chronic schizophrenic with a long history of medication noncompliance that led to 17 hospitalizations in Connecticut, Rhode Island, and California over the past 10 years." This is simply the basic information that the practitioner already knows from the assessments. The question to ask in order to generate a good quality formulation is what is the understanding behind WHY the person chose not to use medications? This is a critical step in the planning process as the answer to the WHY question can bring the practitioner's understanding to a new level, which will have direct implications for how issues are then addressed in the recovery plan.

In the case formulation, the plan writer is challenged to dig deeper and answer the WHY question because depending on the reason behind the person's choice not to use medications, the writer may include very different types of objectives and interventions in the PCCP. For example, a person might have been concerned about side effects such as weight gain and/or disruption of sexual function. Here it would be helpful to take the person, who is concerned about a side-effect of weight gain, for a consultation with a nutritionist or talking with the person about possible plan for increased physical activity to offset weight gain, or exploring alternative medications where weight gain is not as prominent. Or the practitioner might consider family-based interventions if psychiatric medications are interfering with sexual relationships and the person needs support in discussing this with the partner. If an individual is not using meds because he/she does not believe in having an illness or feels the meds are harmful, it might be particularly effective to offer trust-building, motivational psychoeducation and perhaps peer specialist services. Other individuals might have religious or cultural objections and might prefer more faith-based or cultural interventions in managing the illness. In this case, it might be helpful to reach out to someone in the individual's faith-based or cultural community to solicit support regarding preferred healing practices. How does the individual understand his/her experience of symptoms? How can we engage the person in a conversation around his/her illness and recovery? Some individuals may not take medications because their family members have told them not to or made them feel embarrassed about this experience. Some family members, like others in the community, may carry a strong stigma about mental health services and medications and may discourage their loved one from making use of these supports. So this might suggest a need for family education or a referral to NAMI (National Alliance on Mental Illness), for example. Still other individuals might have difficulty organizing their med regimen due to cognitive disabilities or traumatic brain injury or difficulty simply paying for their medications due to insurance and financial issues. Getting to this deeper level of understanding allows the practitioner to then present highly individualized supports that appropriately target the WHY behind an individual's choice not to use medications. Note that this does not mean that the practitioner necessarily abandons their clinical recommendation on the use of medication. It does, however, challenge the practitioner to listen to, and value, a person's lived experience as doing so can lead to a deeper level of understanding, which is reflected in the integrated formulation.

Now that the distinction between assessment data (the WHAT) and the integrated formulation (the WHY) has been made clear, it is important to move to the next step: how is this understanding documented and how is it used in the clinical process? The integrated summary should be recorded in a multi-paragraph narrative, and it should be shared with the person (and the family or other members of the recovery team, if so desired by the individual). This sharing of information is consistent with the notion of transparency and partnership as discussed in Module 2, and should be the norm. Only in rare circumstances (e.g., early in the helping relationship in working with a trauma survivor whose history may be, as yet, outside his or her awareness, or when working with someone with a psychotic disorder who is not yet ready to acknowledge having such a condition) would it be clinically indicated to withhold information. Note that "sharing" of the integrated summary can be done in the form of a written narrative or it can be equally powerful to simply discuss the summary with the individual in a more informal manner, giving them ample opportunity to reflect and add, or even at times correct, the practitioner's understanding.

Being transparent in this manner, as well as checking the validity of the staff person's formulation with the individual, is an important reflection of the mutual respect and partnership on which the PCCP process is built. Simply asking the question "This is how I am seeing you and your situation at this moment, did I get it right?" goes a long way toward trust and relationship building. Insights gained into the nature of the person's difficulties, and their possible solutions, should include some consideration of the diagnosis while also identifying the individual's and family's strengths and resources. The formulation begins to clarify interrelationships between the various facets of the person's life including goals and strengths, as well as barriers and challenges. In doing so, the integrated summary or formulation serves as a bridge between the data of the assessment and the creation of the individualized, person-centered plan.

Preparing an integrated summary or formulation can be a challenge for many staff. And while there is no one agreed on formula, we present an approach drawn from the field of psychiatry and the work of Adams and Grieder [8] to assist the construction of this formulation. The following outline, organized around a set of variables each beginning with the letter "P", includes consideration of:

- *P* ertinent history in *brief*: brief introduction and sketch of the individual's history
- *P* resent condition/presenting problem: description of the current status including experience of symptoms and functional abilities/limitations
- *P* redisposing factors: underlying variables/experiences which may predispose the person to difficulties, e.g., genetic predisposition for mental illness, co-occurring medical issues or cognitive impairments, history of trauma, etc.

- *P* recipitating factors: a description of events or major stressors that led up to a person's decision to seek care
- *P* erpetuating factors: factors which may prolong distress or negative outcomes, e.g., untreated substance use, lack of social supports, chronic medical conditions, etc.
- *P* revious treatment and response: treatments and supports used and how these have helped or hindered recovery in the past

In keeping with the strengths-based and self-directed nature of PCCP, the following "P" variables are given unique attention within the person-centered formulation or integrated summary.

- *P* rioritization by the person served: What goals might the person want to work on now, or later?
- *P* references of the person served: Preferences around treatment options, and life circumstances
- *P* rotective factors: range of strengths, interests, and resources (including natural supports) which may be actively used in the PCCP process

These prompts are suggested here with the understanding that they will not all apply equally to all individuals. For example, at the onset of the problems, understanding the predisposing and precipitating factors may be quite important, while for the ongoing problems, understanding the perpetuating factors might be considered more critical.

Identifying and Prioritizing Goals

It is not uncommon for people to emerge from the assessment and formulation tasks with multiple needs and goals. Prioritization is now the next important step in the logic of building a quality person-centered plan. The average person cannot address all the areas of their life at the same time and will need to focus on what is most important to them in their unique recovery process. Plans with multiple goals, each with multiple objectives and corresponding objectives, are often overwhelming, and efforts are diluted across so many areas that the ultimate result is that sustained progress is not made in any one of them. It is the job of the team to work collaboratively with the individual to prioritize their list of needs so that a manageable number will get attention and the person will have a greater likelihood of making progress.

Throughout the process of prioritization, practitioners must be mindful of balancing what they think is *important FOR* the individual (from their professional perspective) with what might be *important TO* the individual (through the lens of his/her own preferences and values). Sometimes they are the same thing, sometimes they are not. Balancing priorities, and the perspectives of both the practitioner and the person, is a concept that comes out of other disability arenas and it is central to the partnership on which person-centered planning must be based.[1] The important FOR individuals is often where we bring our

---

[1] See "Becoming a Person Centred System": A paper by Michael Smull, Mary Lou Bourne and Helen Sanderson. This can be accessed at http://www.helensandersonassociates.co.uk/whats-new/'becoming-a-person-centred-system'-a-paper-by-michael-smull,-mary-lou-bourne-and-helen-sanderson.aspx

professional perspectives to the table and where we must think about certain core safety and health factors, stabilization of risk issues, legal obligations, and others. Having said that, we also have to consider what is important TO people, that is, the things that make them happy, content, and fulfilled. While practitioners may be focused on stabilizing psychosis, the individual may be motivated to do so only for a particular reason, and that reason – that driving motivation or goal – needs to somehow be reflected in the plan.

Typically, the thing that people most value is enjoying their life in the community, which might involve being a good father, attending church, volunteering at a soup kitchen, taking care of an elderly friend, finishing a GED – whatever it might be, the plan should ultimately be developed with these things in mind. Unfortunately, during the task of prioritization, it is not at all uncommon for the plan to be dominated by those things practitioners feel are *important for* the person, which subsequently become active goals on the plan (e.g., maintaining abstinence, increasing insight, complying with medications as prescribed) whereas those things that are important *to* the person (e.g., moving out of the group home, visiting a grandson, taking a poetry class) are deferred or put off indefinitely. In contrast, adopting a more person-centered approach in planning challenges practitioners to place the individual's valued goals front-and-center in the plan rather than delaying them in the name of striving for "clinical stability."

Despite their best efforts at collaboration, there will be times where practitioners and persons in recovery do not see eye to eye, and they may find themselves in situations where they need to agree to disagree. For example, if a practitioner feels there is a core risk and safety issue, even if the person states they are unwilling to address it, it may need to be discussed and addressed in the treatment plan in some manner, for example, by documenting that the practitioner has shared his/her concerns and suggestions so that the person can make a decision informed not only by their personal preferences but also by sound clinical recommendations. In circumstances where there is disagreement, however, it is important for the practitioner to also remember their obligation to continue to use their best-practice motivational and engagement strategies, and to truly understand what is important to the person and what his or her perspective is on the issue at hand.

Striking this balance in perspectives has been referred to by Patricia Deegan, an internationally renowned teacher and researcher in the recovery movement, as finding the common ground or the "Recovery Zone." Person-centered planning is not just about handing the keys over to the individual and letting them be in the driver's seat while disregarding clinical concerns. For example, if a person wants to abruptly stop the medications, which we know has had disastrous consequences in the past, practitioners should not simply look the other way in the name of honoring the person's choice, abandoning them to the consequences of their choice. This is not person-centered planning. This is sheer *neglect*. At the other end of the spectrum, it is also not advisable to go behind closed doors and strategize about how the team is going to get the individual to do the thing they want them to do without involving the person in the dialogue. This is not person-centered planning. This is *coercion*. Person-centered planning is based more on a partnership model and it challenges practitioners and service users to find that common ground of the Recovery Zone.

In summary, the balancing of professional and personal perspectives is critical at all phases of the PCCP process, and is particularly important during the task of setting priorities as this sets the stage for the "core" focus of the care plan that is described in the following section.

Additional Tools and Resources

Sample Strengths-Based, Person-Centered Inquiry

Rationale: Focusing solely on deficits in the absence of a thoughtful analysis of strengths disregards the most critical resources an individual has on which to build in his or her efforts to advance in his or her recovery. Therefore, the assessment of strengths and resources, including how they might inform the treatment plan, is an essential component of person-centered recovery planning. This assessment should be completed through discussions with the individual, and (with the individual's permission) through collateral contacts with the individual's family and natural supports.

Introduction: Today I am going to be asking you a lot of questions so I can get to know you better. Some of the questions might be things like: What do you like to do for fun?, Who are the most important people in your life?, What are your dreams for the future? You may won-der what all of these questions have to do with your mental health or with your treatment here at _____. And that would be a great question. We think that these things can, or should be, a very important part of your recovery and treatment. Because sometimes the best way to deal with symptoms or things we struggle with is by using our strengths or things we are good at. Together, we'll learn more about those things, and also talk a bit about how you might put them into action and include them in your recovery plan.

A: Interests and Activities

A1. What does your "typical" day look like?
A2. Are there ways that you could improve your day or make it more enjoyable?
A3. What activities/hobbies do you enjoy at home? In the community?
A4. Who do you enjoy these things with?
A5. If you could plan the "perfect day," what would it look like?

B: Living Environment

B1. Describe where you currently live?
B2. How satisfied are you with this living arrangement?
B3. What do you like best about it? What would make it better?
B4. Are you interested in living in another place? If so, what setting would you prefer?
B5. What are the most important things to you when deciding where to live?
B6. What would make your living space feel more "homey" … ?

C: Employment

C1. Are you currently working? If so, where? What do you do? Is it full-time or part-time?
C2. How do you feel about your job?
C3. Do you do any volunteer work? If so, where? What do you do?
C4. Have you worked in the past? If so, what type of positions have you held?
C5. What did you like the most about those jobs?

C6. What did you like the least about those jobs?
C7. What would be your ideal job? Think back to the time before you first began to struggle (before the hospitalizations, etc.), what did you dream of being when you grew up and why?

D: Learning

D1. What was school like for you?
D2. What was your favorite subject?
D3. What kinds of things have you studied or learned in the past? In school or in other types of learning groups, for example, book clubs, bible study?
D4. What would you like to learn now?

E: Safety and Legal Issues

E1. Are you dealing with any legal issues right now?
E2. If your legal issues are bothering you, how can your team help?

F: Financial

F1. What are your sources of income?
F2. Does anyone help you with money management? If so, how do they help you?
F3. What do you spend your money on? What do you do to stretch your dollars?
F4. How much control do you have in managing your money? How is that working for you?
F5. Would you like to be more independent with managing your finances? If so, how do you think you could do that? Who could help you?

G: Lifestyle and Health

G1. What do you do to take care of your health?
G2. Do you have any concerns about your overall health?
G3. Are you getting enough rest? Are you getting enough exercise? Are you interested in exercising more?
G4. Are you satisfied with the amount and kinds of foods you eat? Are you interested in changing your diet?
G5. Are there other habits you'd like to change? If so, what kind of help would you need?
G6. Now, can you tell me a little bit specifically about your mental health? How have things been going for you lately?
G7. Have you had any concerns about your medication? Do you feel like they are helping you? Are you being bothered by any side effects?
G8. How does your family and/or community respond to your mental health challenges?
G9. How does your family feel about you taking medications? What would you like for them to know?
G10. What kinds of services have you received in the past to help you manage your symptoms and your recovery?
G11. And how helpful have you found these services to be?
G12. Do these programs/services make you feel comfortable as a person?

G13. Do you think your therapist addresses your cultural issues? If so, how does he or she do this? If not, how could he or she do this, meaning what would you like for him/her to do differently?

G14. Are there things you do on your own that help you feel better?

H: Transportation

H1. How do you get around town?

H2. Would you like to expand your options for getting around, for example, learning the bus routes?

H3. Who could help you do this?

I: Personal Strengths

I1. My best qualities as a person are …

I2. Something I would NOT change about myself is …

I3. I am most proud of …

I4. My sense of humor is …

I5. The times I am most at peace are when …

I6. People like that I am (people say they like my …)

I7. The things that help me to make it through the day when I am down are …

I8. I help other people out by … (Something I give to others that makes me feel good is …)

I11. My heroes are …

I12. I feel I am doing better when …

J: Choice-Making

J1. Do you feel like you can stand up for yourself? If so, how do you stand up for yourself?

J2. What are some of the choices that you currently have made in your life?

J3. Are there choices in your life that are made for you? If yes, tell us a bit more about that …

J4. How does it make you feel to have others make choices for you?

J5. If other people make choices for you, does it give you a sense of security? How does it make you feel?

J6. Do you have an Advance Directive [explain as needed]? If so, is your primary clinician/case manager aware of it and how best to honor it in the event of a crisis situation?

K: Faith and Spirituality

K1. How important is faith/spirituality in your life?

K2. What type of spiritual or faith activities do you participate in?

K3. How satisfied are you with your opportunities to participate in your spiritual practice or attend the congregation of your choice right now?

K4. How/What kind of help do you need to help you find the spiritual support you are seeking or to participate in a religious community (if it is clear that the person is seeking this support)?

K5. Are there people in your church or faith community who are aware of your mental health challenges? How has that been helpful to or hindered your recovery?

L: Relationships

L1. Who are the most important people in your life right now?
L2. Is there someone who believes in you?
L3. Do you feel understood?
L5. When you need someone to talk to or lean on, who do you turn to?
L6. [For persons of color] Do you have other people of color role models with mental health challenges that you can talk to? Is this something you would like?
L7. Are there people who depend on you?
L8. What do you look for in a close relationship?
L9. What kinds of qualities do you bring to a relationship?
L10. Do you have a romantic or intimate relationship?
L11. How is it going?
L12. Are you satisfied with your sexual life?
L13. Why or why not?
L14. Is there anyone you'd like to spend more time with?

M: Hopes and Dreams

M1. Could you tell me a bit about your hopes or dreams for the future?
M2. Have your hopes and dreams changed over time? If so, how?
M3. What kinds of dreams did you have before you started having mental health difficulties?
M4. How did they change and why?
N5. When you were a child, what did you want to become when you grew up?
M6. What are some things in your life that you hope you can do and change in the future?
M7. Do you feel like you are able to do those things or make those changes?
M8. If you went to bed and a miracle happened while you were sleeping, what would be different when you woke up? How would you know things were different?

Exercises

Exercise 1. Consider the following questions regarding strengths.

1. What is gained when we explore, uncover, identify, and include strengths and wellness activities in the recovery planning process?
2. How might identification with a cultural or social or spiritual group help promote wellness?
3. How might we, as providers, promote that identification even though it might not be part of our service delivery system?
4. What are 3 of your strengths?
5. What are 3 of your skills?
6. What are 3 of your talents?
7. Now for a bit of reflection: how was it to answer the previous three questions? Easy? Hard?
8. How does identifying your own strengths inform (if at all) your work with people receiving services?

Exercise 2. Roma: An example for person-centered planning.

Read the below example of Roma. Roma's story is presented with information you would need to create a comprehensive person-centered formulation as described throughout this Module. Feel free to add whatever additional information you need. After reading through Roma's assessment data create your own integrated formulation. Compare it to the sample provided and assess the extent to which you feel you included the following dimensions, does the narrative:

- Present an individualized picture?
- Identify strengths?
- Describe functional impairments (i.e., symptoms are not listed in a vacuum)?
- Include role of natural supports if any?
- Note any cultural factors that may impact treatment and recovery?
- Describe the stage of change?
- Present an integrated understanding/hypothesis regarding the individual's difficulties?

History, demographics, and presenting issue

Roma is a 29-year-old, Puerto Rican female who has been treated on and off in the New Haven system of care for 15 years due to problems associated with her diagnosis of major depression, posttraumatic stress disorder, and poly-substance abuse. She was incarcerated from 2008 to 2009 for drug-related offenses (possession of heroin, theft, prostitution) and risk of injury to a minor (repeated driving while intoxicated with children in her car; leaving children unattended during drug binges). During this time, her children (a 14-year-old daughter and a 9-year-old son) were in the custody of her cousin who is a supportive influence in Roma's life and recovery. Following her release from prison 4 months ago, Roma was referred to *outpatient mental health* and *addiction services* and began living with her cousin and her kids. However, she started drinking and then stole several of her cousin's prescription medications including Vicodin and Xanax. Once, the cousin had left the kids overnight in Roma's care to attend an out-of-state funeral. When she returned, she found that Roma had passed out on the couch and she had no idea where her 9-year-old was. It turned out that the 9-year-old was playing basketball at the local community court, and Roma later admitted that she had left the kids alone the night before to go out and buy drugs. In addition, Roma's cousin says that Roma had been having great difficulty setting limits with the children, and that she relates to them more as a friend than as a maternal figure. In addition, there were frequent verbal "blowouts" with her teenage daughter, and on one occasion, Roma slapped her across the face when she was high. Roma's cousin is very concerned about Roma's continued drug use and her volatile relationship with her daughter, so she asked Roma to leave the apartment until she "cleaned up her act."

Child protective services have been involved in Roma's case for several years given her previous charges and difficulties taking care of the kids. When Roma had to leave her cousin's apartment, her protective services case worker suggested she seek temporary housing and services at a homeless shelter. She has been at the shelter for 3 weeks now, and she makes it clear that she wants to work toward regaining custody of her children with the help of her mental health providers and her shelter case manager. Her cousin is willing to let Roma visit the kids provided that Roma is taking steps to get her life back on track. According to conditions outlined in her probation order and her protective services mandates, Roma must engage in mental health and addictions treatment, secure stable housing, pursue employment or disability benefits for financial security, and demonstrate adequate parenting skills before she can regain the legal custody of her children.

Family background/early childhood

Born in Puerto Rico, Roma is the fourth child. Her mother reportedly suffered from serious mental illness and abandoned the children when Roma was 6 years old. She was then raised by her maternal grandmother for 2 years until the age of 8 when the grandmother passed away suddenly. She moved in with her biological father, who began an incestuous relationship with Roma, which lasted until Roma became pregnant by him at the age of 14. Roma ran away from home, and with the help of neighbors, she contacted her extended family in the United States and relocated to New York to live with a maternal aunt and uncle. The aunt and uncle are now deceased, but Roma continues to be close with her cousin who currently has legal custody of her children.

Education/employment

After relocating to the United States, Roma enrolled in high school while her aunt and uncle assisted with child care responsibilities for her daughter. She was an average student, but an avid reader who also excelled in creative writing and arts classes. However, she quickly became involved in a number of abusive relationships, and turned to drugs and alcohol as she became increasingly depressed. Roma dropped out of school mid-way in her junior year. She has worked on and off as a housecleaner for the past decade; however, mental health issues and substance abuse, as well as an additional pregnancy (from a brief relationship), have made it difficult for her to finish school or maintain a job for any period of time. While at the shelter, she has shown responsibilities with chores around the program and, under the supervision of one of the shelter staff, has been volunteering to help with some clerical and reception tasks.

Health status

Recently, Roma has been diagnosed with early-stage cirrhosis of the liver secondary to years of alcohol abuse.

Mental health symptoms and treatment

Roma has undergone times when she had been so depressed that she had recurrent thoughts of suicide. On two occasions (over 5 years ago), she took an overdose of her medications, which led to both medical and psychiatric hospitalization. Currently, Roma denies suicidal ideation, and she has been using her medications effectively to alleviate her symptoms. Despite this, she reports that her "nerves" continue to cause her great distress. She has severe sleep disturbances (unable to sleep through the night due to nightmares) and is sometimes too depressed and exhausted to get out of bed in the morning. This has made it very difficult for her to look for work or an apartment as she is feeling very overwhelmed. In addition, she admits to being irritable and having volatile interpersonal relationships, especially with her daughter, with whom she has frequent verbal (and on one occasion, physical) altercations.

Alcohol/drug use

Roma has abused marijuana, heroin, and prescription drugs, but for the past 10 years, her primary drug has been alcohol. When drinking, her judgment can be significantly impaired (e.g., she has left her children unattended) and her behavior can be aggressive (e.g., she was arrested in 2001 for assaulting her then-boyfriend with a broken vodka bottle). Despite previous criminal charges and the current involvement of child protective services, Roma tends to minimize her alcohol and drug use stating that she needed to drink to "numb out" as she could not handle the stress of her life. While Roma has not had any positive toxicology screens reported by her clinician, she does admit to "slips" and her cousin reports that her attendance at Alcoholics Anonymous and Narcotics Anonymous meetings has dropped off in the past two months. Roma herself admits to having increased cravings, but says she has been clean since staying at the shelter and seems motivated to stay sober and to find alternative, healthy ways to manage stress.

Strengths, interests, and goals

Roma is in the active stage of change in relation to her use of alcohol and other drugs. She is motivated to make progress in her recovery and put her "life back together." She recognizes the need to replace her drinking and drug use with positive stress management strategies. She is also a deeply loving mother who has managed, with the support of her cousin, to provide for her children through the years despite a serious trauma history and subsequent mental health and addiction issues. She has a strong desire to improve her relationship with her children and wants to be a better role model for them. She is well liked by other clients at the shelter and has done well as a volunteer in the reception area where she has been answering phones and directing guests. Throughout her struggles in life, Roma has always "escaped" through painting as well as reading and writing poetry. She is highly creative and enjoys all forms of artistic expression. She hopes to finish high school and someday find work in an environment where she can be around books or artists.

Keeping in mind the material presented in this module, create, on a separate page of paper, a sample integrated formulation for Roma that balances the presentation of her needs with an emphasis on her strengths and resources. When you are finished, compare your integrated summary to the one provided here.

Sample Formulation

Roma is a 29-year-old Puerto Rican woman, and a deeply loving mother of a daughter (age 14) and a son (age 9). She has, at times through the years, relied on the support of her cousin to provide for her children as she struggled to manage a serious trauma history and subsequent mental health (major depression and PTSD) and addiction issues (poly-substance abuse). Roma's cousin has been a stable and supportive influence for many years, including taking care of her daughter at times when she has been unable to do so herself. She was recently referred to your rehab agency by her clinic therapist and her Child Protective Services case worker after she was asked to leave her cousin's apartment due to what her cousin refers to as her "destructive behaviors" and inability to parent her children. In particular, Roma was having increasing difficulty relating to her 14-year-old daughter and managing her behavior and this lead to frequent volatile arguments. This pattern may have been due in part to irritability associated with depression and Roma's intermittent alcohol use; however, the daughter is currently at the same age that Roma was when she became pregnant with her as a result of sexual abuse and incest at the hands of her father. It is possible that this is triggering an increase in trauma-related stress and symptoms, and making it particularly difficult for Roma to effectively parent her daughter.

Roma has been living in your Transitional Housing Program for 3 weeks now, and while she is feeling very overwhelmed and distressed by her situation and by persistent symptoms, she is hopeful regarding the program and what it has to offer. She has a number of strengths and interests she can draw on in her recovery. She is a devoted parent who has demonstrated significant resilience having survived multiple traumas and losses in her life. Consistent with her culture of origin, she places a high value on family support, has benefitted from a close relationship with her cousin, and may prefer natural supports to formal treatment services. Roma is also highly creative and artistic and has found refuge in painting, which she uses as a coping skill. She has made it clear that her priority goal is to work toward regaining custody of her children, and she is in the action stage of change and motivated to work with her clinic therapist, her Residential Counselor, and other Outreach Workers in order to develop the stability and skills needed to be the best mother she can be.

Learning Assessment

Module 4: Strength-based Assessment, Integrated Understanding, and Setting Priorities		
Statement	True	False
1. A discussion of strengths should be the central focus of every assessment, care plan, and case summary.		
2. Person-centered care planning means the person needs to make his or her own decisions without input from anyone else other than the mental health professionals involved in his or her care.		
3. Strength-based assessment means disregarding the needs and focusing solely on the strengths and capacities.		
4. Spirituality and sexuality are areas that should be explored in person-centered assessments.		
5. Personal autonomy, self-determination, and independence may be values inconsistent with an individual's cultural worldview.		
See the Answer Key at the end of the chapter for the correct answers. **Number Correct**		
0 to 2: You have a lot to learn, but we hope you find this guide useful in the process! 3 to 4: You have a solid foundation. Use this guide to enhance your skills and the supports you offer. 5: You are ahead of the game! Use this guide to teach others and strive for excellence.		

References

1. Tondora J, Pocklington S, Gregory GA *et al.* (2005) *Implementation of Person-Centered Care and Planning: How Philosophy can Inform Practice*. Substance Abuse and Mental Health Services Administration, Rockville, MD.
2. Rapp CA. (1998) *The Strengths Model: Case Management with People Suffering from Severe and Persistent Mental Illness*. Oxford University Press, New York.
3. Saleeby D. (2001) The diagnostics strengths manual. *Social Work* **46**, 183–187.
4. DeJong P, Miller SD. (1995) How to interview for clients' strengths. *Social Work* **40**, 729–736.
5. Cowger CD. (1994). Assessing clients' strengths: Clinical assessment for client empowerment. *Social Work* **39**, 262–268.
6. American Psychiatric Association. (2000) *Diagnostic and Statistical Manual for Mental Disorders*. 4th edition, text revision. American Psychiatric Association, Washington, DC.

7. Humphreys S, Townsend W. (2005) *The Impact of Culture on Person/Family Centered Planning*. Paper presented at the person/family centered planning consensus conference, December 8th, Washington, DC.
8. Adams N, Grieder D. (2005) *Treatment Planning for Person-Centered Care: The road to Mental Health and Addiction Recovery*. Elsevier Academic Press, San Diego, CA.

Answers to the Learning Assessment:

1. T
2. F
3. F
4. T
5. T

Module 5: Creating the plan through a team meeting

Goal

This module introduces the "nuts and bolts" of actually creating a plan with a focus on the team meeting and helping the individual to assure that all of the right people are involved in a quality person-centered process.

Learning Objectives

After completing this module, you should be better able to:

- describe the roles and responsibilities of team members;
- identify at least five key indicators of a well-run PCCP meeting;
- identify a wide range of both professional and community supports who can contribute to PCCP, including peer supporters.

Learning Assessment

A knowledge-learning assessment is included at the end of the module. If you are already familiar with the planning process, you may want to go to the end of this module and take the assessment test to see how much you know already. Then you can focus your learning efforts on the materials that are new for you.

The preplanning activities presented in Modules 3 and 4 offer critical information about how practitioners can help to elicit the individual's goals, strengths, personal and cultural preferences, and network of supporters. These details should be organized and readily available to inform the subsequent planning meeting and its various steps and procedures, beginning with determining who should attend the planning meeting.

Partnering for Recovery in Mental Health: A Practical Guide to Person-Centered Planning, First Edition.
Janis Tondora, Rebecca Miller, Mike Slade and Larry Davidson.
© 2014 John Wiley & Sons, Ltd. Published 2014 by John Wiley & Sons, Ltd.

Determining Who Should Attend

Practitioners should help the person to identify people who he or she believes will consider his or her best interest. In order to decide who should be invited to the meeting, practitioners should encourage the individual to think about the following:

- Who among your family and friends understand your pathway to recovery and what will help you to progress on your way? Who has offered helpful support in the past?
- Person-centered care plans (PCCPs) consider not only what you *need* from your team and the mental health system, but how you, in turn, can *give back* to others. Who knows your gifts and talents, and encourages you to use them to make meaningful contributions to the community, for example, through advocacy, employment, or volunteering?
- Who would feel comfortable speaking in the meeting in an honest and responsible way? Keep in mind that it may take time for some people to be active, vocal participants as their efforts to help in the past may have been rejected by you or other team members.
- Individuals who know the community and its resources and who are sensitive to your cultural identity can be very important contributors in the meeting. Have a conversation with these individuals to let them know why you would like them to be a part of your support network, what you know about the process, and what you believe will be expected of them. Ask them to play a part in your care planning process.
- You may use the Circle of Supports exercise (see Module 3) to identify the people you would like to invite to join your planning team. Remember, you may want to include friends, family, service providers, neighbors, the clerk at the store who helps you with your shopping each week, your teacher, or anyone else you choose.
- Remember that the team can, and often should, change over time based on how your goals change over time. For example, you may initially choose to have only a close friend and one direct service provider involved. Over time, you may find that your family has an important role to play. Or perhaps you have just returned to work and a job coach or a coworker might make helpful contributions. The composition of the team can change at any time. Not all decisions need to be made now!

Care planning can be far more successful if the individual involves people who are important in his or her life. One function of the practitioner can be to help the individual to identify these existing supports (through the kinds of questions noted above) or to help the individual to develop new ones in cases where such supports do not currently exist. For example, a care plan can include a fellow parishioner who offers to provide rides to Sunday services or to be a companion at a weekly Bible Study group. Creative use of community supports and spreading out support tasks are some of the highly desirable features of PCCPs. However, it is also possible that an individual may not wish to have others involved in the planning process due to personal or cultural preferences. People can be educated about the potential benefit of involving others, but this is always a matter of choice and is done only at the person's request.

Ideally, these activities will lead to an initial meeting that involves people who know and care about the individual, including a mix of staff, advocates, family members, and friends. At this meeting, information regarding the goals and structure of the planning session will be reviewed and all attendees will have an opportunity to ask questions. This process builds on the pre-meeting orientation and education discussed in Module 3. Reviewing this orientation, at least briefly, is essential, as all meeting participants need to be clear on the purpose and format of the planning sessions.

Setting the Logistics of the Meeting

Once the individual has some idea of who she or he would like to invite to be a part of the planning team meeting, the next step is identifying the time and location of the first (or next) meeting. A simple, yet powerful, strategy is ensuring that the individual has advance notification of this planning meeting as well as reasonable control over the meeting logistics, for example, what time the meeting takes place and who is invited to participate. All too often individuals arrive at their regular sessions or appointments and are notified that their treatment plan is overdue so "today is the day we need to get that on the books." Given the importance of the decisions made in person-centered planning meetings, this lack of advance notice can place an unreasonable burden on the person to be prepared to launch into a discussion of their most valued hopes, dreams, and desires—as well as the difficult issues that may have been getting in the way. In such circumstances, it is not uncommon for the person to clam up, or for the practitioner and the person together to just default to a cookie-cutter, "business as usual" treatment plan that has little individualization and recovery focus. Wherever possible, giving people advance information, for example, "It is that time of year again when we will need to be updating your recovery plan together. If it's OK with you, I'd like to try to schedule that for 2 weeks from now, and in the meantime, I'd like you to be thinking about what kinds of goals you'd like to focus on in the coming months and what kinds of steps we might need to take to help you reach those goals. And, of course, if there is anyone you'd like to invite—a family member, a friend—just let me know and we will do what we can to arrange a meeting time that works for everyone on the team."

This last element highlights the importance of the individual having a *reasonable* degree of input into the logistics of the planning meeting. Note the emphasis on the term "reasonable." We are not suggesting that in person-centered planning, individuals can dictate that they can come, for example, only on the third Tuesday of the month at 3 PM as that is the only time their spouse is available! That would go beyond what would be considered "reasonable" input. However, consider how you make important medical appointments in your own life—particularly those where you might like the support of a family member or friend. In such cases, you might request, for example, "It's very important to me that my husband be there with me to be a part of the discussion because he is a very important part of my decision making. So, if at all possible, if we can try to schedule the meeting later in the afternoon, that would make it much more likely that he will be able to be there to support me." It is this type of courtesy in scheduling that we might expect in arranging our own health care appointments, and in person-centered planning, we work hard to honor this same accommodation.

The individual or plan facilitator (who may, or may not, be the primary clinical practitioner, see below) should notify the potential team members of the meeting date, time, place, and agenda well in advance. While efforts should be made to ensure that the focus person will be as comfortable as possible, the time and place of the meeting need to meet the convenience of other attendees as well. Some individuals prefer the meeting at their home, while some would rather have the meeting at a neutral place such as a room at an office. Team meetings can be held at diners or coffee shops if privacy can be assured. While there are no defined rules regarding the structure and logistics of the meeting, the overarching goal is to allow the person to set priorities and to have reasonable control over the date, time, and place of his/her PCCP meeting. The practitioner assists and supports the individual in making these arrangements.

While team-based planning should occur at a time most conducive to the maximum number of team participants being present, there will inevitably be times when an important person will not be able to attend. Practitioners should make every effort to adjust the schedules and times so that as many team members as possible can be included. It is vital to remember that a team member can be on the team and not in the meeting, if their input is solicited prior to the meeting and if they are briefed after the meeting. Sometimes team members also participate by phone or via a computer link.

Respectful Team Meetings: Starting with the Basics

There are some basic respectful practices in the treatment team process that we should be aware of as a starting point to ensure the PCCP meeting is maximally responsive to the person's needs and preferences. These practices should be followed automatically though they are not yet a part of standard practice.

- Team members should arrive on time for the meeting as it can be disconcerting and disruptive for participants to be coming and going throughout the discussion.
- The meeting facilitator should ensure that all members introduce themselves and their role in the focus person's life. This is particularly critical when new members, such as natural supporters, are joining the team for the first time.
- It is important to ensure that you are giving the person your full attention by turning off cell phones, not having side bar conversations, and not charting in their, or someone else's, medical record, while the person is present and the team is engaged in conversation. Think of this as a fully protected time for the person in recovery!
- Be cognizant of the tendency to talk about the person (as if she or he is not in the room) rather than talking directly with them. Questions/comments should first be directed to him or her (e.g., asking them how they think their groups are going and if they are making progress) rather than soliciting this information only from the staff member/group leader. When teams are feeling pressured for time to get through all the necessary agenda items, it can seem easier and quicker to ask questions of staff; but remember, we are striving for more of a partnership and a balance of perspectives.

Defining Roles and Responsibilities of Team Members

Each member of the care planning team has a unique role to fulfill in the planning and plan oversight process, but everyone involved is there to support the individual and his/her recovery priorities. Table 5.1 [1] summarizes the roles of respective team members and additional information is provided here.

The Role and Responsibilities of the PCCP Facilitator

What is a PCCP facilitator, and what role does the facilitator play? The "facilitator" is someone who is trained in, and committed to, the principles and practices of PCCP. In other disciplines and fields, such as the developmental disabilities field, there may be independent facilitators who act as the coordinator of the process. In the mental health systems with which we have worked, this setup has not been feasible because of time and fiscal pressures. Most commonly, the primary clinician or practitioner is the organizer and facilitator of the meeting. Therefore, in this document, we refer to the meeting leader as the clinician or practitioner. This is in no way to discount the role of the independent facilitator as it works in other PCCP models, but more so in recognition of the current practice of many mental health systems and the limited feasibility of having an outside facilitator.

An additional possibility is to have a peer specialist act as the coordinator or facilitator of the meeting. META Services Recovery Education Center of Phoenix, for example, employs "recovery coaches" as facilitators of PCCP meetings. A central function of the Recovery Coach is to assist individuals in completing a *Self-Directed Recovery Plan* and to provide peer support as the individual works on his or her plan for recovery. Expanding the role of peer specialist employees to include PCCP facilitation is a particularly promising practice, and research is underway to assess its effectiveness.

Within the PCCP meeting, the practitioner works to ensure that the values and steps of the process are delivered in a manner that is consistent with PCCP's fundamental principles. The following list notes the essential skills for running such a meeting:

Listening skills:

- Being able to listen to what people are "saying" (in overt verbal language as well as subtle body language).
- Being able to assist team members to listen to each other.
- Being able to listen below the surface to what is not being said.

Visioning skills:

- Being able to think, and assist others to think, beyond the formal service system to include a network of natural supports.
- Being able to assist the person receiving services and the planning team members to dream big!
- Being able to suggest large and small dreams, goals, and objectives.
- Being able to work with the team to tap into community supports and activities.
- Being able to solicit information from team members such as how to access culturally appropriate services.
- Being able to encourage the person receiving services to use gifts and skills to further his or her own recovery *and* to give back to team members or the community as a whole.

Table 5.1   Roles and Responsibilities of PCCP Team Members

Focus Person (for whom the plan is being developed)	Facilitator	Family (as defined by individual) and other supports (including community representatives)
Has the leadership role in developing the plan. Has ownership of the plan. May or may not select the facilitator for the planning process. Is responsible for full participation in the process. Thinks about and communicates his or her hopes, dreams, desires, needs, likes, dislikes, and so on as clearly as possible using whatever means appropriate to his or her abilities. Expects the facilitator, practitioners, family members, and other natural supporters to work *with* him or her, not *for* him or her. Builds relationships with planning team members. Is willing to be creative and take responsibility and risks to achieve his or her stated goals. Stays committed to the process.	*Embraces all responsibilities common to other attendees in addition to the following:* Is an advocate for the focus person. Is able to work with team members in an informal way. Provides unconditional support to the person throughout the process. Adjusts the level of facilitation and support as needed based on the person's preferences and current abilities. Encourages the focus person to be as active and empowered as is possible and preferred. Uses "person-centered" and "person-first" language and encourages others to do the same. Helps clarify and communicate the person's ideas to members of the team. Encourages the person to be creative in his or her plan and to take action, responsibility, and responsible risks.	*Common responsibilities include:* Believes in and values the person-directed planning process. Listens to, understands, values, and respects the person in recovery and his or her supporters. Is honest and open in communicating his or her own perspective. Treats all members of the team with respect. Assists the focus person to identify his or her strengths and needs, and to formulate his or her wishes, hopes, dreams, concerns, and so on. Shares knowledge and perspective regarding what has worked and not worked well for the person in the past. Uses "person-first" language. Follows through on agreed-on tasks. Helps to identify and/or pursue resources available to the person from the team or broader community.

Table 5.1   (*continued*)

Focus Person (for whom the plan is being developed)	Facilitator	Family (as defined by individual) and other supports (including community representatives)
	Guides the planning process, keeping everyone and everything focused on the person's wants, needs, desires, dreams, and hopes for his or her life.	Views upsets and disappointments as opportunities to learn, grow, and try new strategies for goal attainment.
	Ensures that all perspectives are heard and given due respect.	Believes in the person's ability to have a positive impact on others and suggests ways in which he or she may do so.
	Uses various tools to help individuals share their story of recovery.	Stays committed to the process.
	Uses consensus-building skills.	Community members also pledge to facilitate the person's pathway to community activities of his or her choice by promoting welcoming and accommodating environments that encourage inclusion.
	Is able to use various means of conflict resolution to manage disputes and/or breakdowns in the planning process.	
	Maintains a record of the planning process.	
	Assists planning team to view and use upsets and disappointments as opportunities to be creative and try new strategies for goal attainment.	
	Reviews and evaluates the process in partnership with the focus person and others as appropriate.	

Adapted from Ref. [1].

Communication:

- Being able to use and to teach others to use person-first language.
- Being able to define and discuss all aspects of PCCP.
- Being able to use common language in place of professional jargon.

Meeting process:

- Being able to assist team members to adhere to PCCP principles throughout the meeting.
- Being able to encourage the person receiving services to be an active participant in the meeting and in the action steps of the plan itself.
- Being able to solicit all viewpoints and to make sure all team members have an opportunity to provide inputs and be heard.
- Being able to build consensus among team members.
- Being able to deal with challenging team members, and to use conflict management skills to deal with conflict.
- Being able to engage team members and to reconvene the group over time as necessary.
- Being able to redirect team members from talking "about" the person receiving services to talking "with" him or her. In some instances, team members may slip into speaking about someone in the third person, almost as if the person is not there. It is the responsibility of the practitioner to redirect and refocus the meeting to be one of collaboration and inclusiveness for the person receiving care.
- Being able to contribute to the development of a collaborative atmosphere in which the focus person is encouraged to take on as much leadership as is preferred and possible.
- Being able to share clinical expertise regarding strategies that might assist the individual in reaching his or her goals.
- Being able to suggest clinical interventions as well as community resources that can potentially assist the individual in reaching important goals.
- Being able to assure compliance with state rules and regulations regarding the delivery of services and supports.
- Being able to attend to the funders' requirements of medical necessity and to allowances under identified billing codes.
- Being able to document the focus person's diagnosis *after* having a transparent discussion with the individual, soliciting his or her perspective, and providing clear explanation when necessary. This discussion can happen during, or prior to, the planning meeting depending on the person's preference.
- Being able to identify the responsibilities and time lines for tasks assumed by each member of the team: service users, advocates, family, friends, community collaborators, and other practitioners or services.
- Being able to draft and review the plan with the focus person and offer the person an opportunity to correct, clarify, or add to the written plan.

> *Y*ou keep talking about getting me in the "driver's seat" of my treatment and my life … when half the time I am not even in the damn car!
>
> —Person in Recovery on her typical role in planning [2]

Periodically, there may be a breakdown in the planning process. If that occurs, the practitioner must enable the group to stay focused, supportive, and on task. The planning process might break down, before, during, after, or completely independent of, a planning meeting. Differences in opinion during the planning meeting can deflect the attention of the team and even derail it. Managing tension and conflict is a key element of leading an effective meeting. While the practitioner who is facilitating pays particular attention to this issue, *every* team member must agree to the respectful treatment of all members of the team. Problem solving and conflict resolution strategies can be helpful tools in these situations, although outlining these is beyond the scope of this manual.[1]

The Role and Responsibilities of the Person Receiving Services

The person receiving services is encouraged to take on a leadership role to the extent that is possible and preferred. There is also an expectation that the person will develop relationships with team members and communicate what he or she needs from them as well as how he or she would like to give back to others in a meaningful way. However, it is recognized that the level of participation and leadership in the planning meeting can be influenced by factors such as cultural values, personal preferences, and the need for skill development. In addition, being in "the driver's seat" may be an intimidating and uncomfortable position for many people who have rarely been in the "damn car" (i.e., the planning meeting) in the past.

The leadership role in PCCP may differ significantly from previous roles people have played in planning their own care, for example, learned helplessness may lead a person to fall back on a more passive role. Finally, individuals may be at a difficult place in their recovery where what is comfortable and preferred is to allow trusted practitioners or natural supporters to take a more directive role until such point as they feel capable of doing so for themselves. This can happen for a variety of reasons including acute distress due to life stressors or symptoms. The challenge to the practitioner and all team members is to meet the person where he or she is "at" (emotionally, cognitively, and culturally) and to adjust the level of support as circumstances change over time, *all the while being careful to respect the person's right to self-direct to the maximum extent possible*. For some individuals, the ability to lead the planning process may come over time or with experience, but the basic assumption of plan ownership still applies throughout.

The Role and Responsibilities of Family and Other Natural Supporters

The primary responsibilities of family members and friends are to attend and to be open, honest, and responsible participants. This includes a commitment to follow-through when

---

[1] For more information on conflict resolution and problem solving strategies, see *Moving On: A Personal Futures Planning Workbook for Individuals with Brain Injury*, Second Edition [1] or "Direct Support Professional Training Resource Guide: Communication, Problem-Solving and Conflict Resolution" [3].

agreeing to certain support tasks. Often, it is family members who have a historical and deep-rooted familiarity with the person's background, dreams, successes, and disappointments. In many cases, where individuals have been unable to get their needs met in the mental health system, they have relied heavily on, and survived based on, the support and care of family members. This intimate family perspective and experience should be received with due respect even if it differs from the views of other members of the team. It is important to allow the focus person to define who he or she would consider a part of his or her "family." This may not be limited to "blood relatives" and may include other close friends and supporters who have an in-depth understanding of the person's past, present, and future dreams and disappointments.

The focus person may also choose to invite an individual from his or her network *not* for the help that he or she can necessarily bring to the process, but because the focus person wishes to "give back" to him or her in a certain way. For example, a person may wish to invite a pastor because he or she would like to discuss starting a Sunday school program in which he or she would be the volunteer teacher. In these circumstances, it is important that the person's desire to give back be respected and that all members of the team believe in the individual's ability to positively impact the lives of others. This type of "reciprocity" in relationships fosters the development of valued social roles and is often a cornerstone of the recovery process [4].

Community acquaintances who are invited to participate in the planning team pledge to support the focus person's wishes to pursue meaningful community activities by striving to create welcoming and accommodating environments. A pastor may provide parish space for the Sunday school program, an employer may connect the individual to a coworker for car-pooling assistance, a college teacher may offer lecture notes in alternative formats (e.g., through readymade outlines or audiotapes), and a friend of the family may invite the person to enroll in his or her pottery class. When given the opportunity and encouragement, natural supporters and other community members can bring meaningful ideas and resources that creatively support the individual's recovery.

The Role and Responsibilities of Administrators

Recognition that the planning process takes organizational efforts and staff time is paramount. Administrators/supervisors should provide space, time, and any other resources necessary for planning meetings. For example, in order to fill the roles and responsibilities noted in this section successfully, all team members must have access to initial training and ongoing coaching regarding PCCP principles and practices. Supervisors and administrators should regularly sit in to observe how PCCP teams are functioning so that they can address organizational barriers and provide feedback and support to staff and other team members as necessary. Organizing additional orientation and training sessions, developing resource manuals, or setting aside time for peer or co-supervision groups can all be effective strategies to promote the quality implementation of PCCP.

Exercises

Exercise 1. Consider the vignette provided below. With three colleagues, role-play Ed's PCCP meeting, keeping in mind the roles and responsibilities reviewed in this module and then discuss the following questions:

1. What was it like for those doing the role play?
2. What did the observers notice?
3. What seems to work?
4. What did not work?
5. How did this role play feel the same/different from planning meetings you are typically involved in? Give examples.
6. What lessons can be taken from this exercise?

Ed's story:

> *Ed used to live in a supervised apartment where his mother, who he is very close to, used to come by frequently for lunch. He also had a close group of young friends (Ed is 22 years old) who he used to enjoy watching football games with on the weekends. According to Ed, these friends always "looked out for him" even when he wasn't "right." However, six months ago, Ed was encouraged by his team to move into a community group home because his health had deteriorated significantly and he was not taking care of his apartment or other important "activities of daily living." The team was worried that Ed's nutritional needs were not being met as Ed has very high-cholesterol and a family history of heart disease and he was not following a physician-prescribed diet. Ed also occasionally missed his medication delivery from his visiting nurse when he was playing pick-up basketball with his friends.*

> *Ed agreed to follow this recommendation of his treatment team and he moved into a community group home. His mother is no longer able to come by on her lunch breaks as the group home expects all residents to be out of the house engaged in productive activity during business hours. His friends can no longer come over for Sunday games, and he has stopped playing pick-up basketball because this involves breaking the curfew of the group home and he is not allowed special treatment. He has lost a few pounds, he is very clean, and so is his apartment—but Ed has made it clear that he is very unhappy and regrets the decision to move to the group home.*

> *Ed recently learned about PCCP from a peer supporter at the mental health center. He has asked for a meeting of his team to make a transition plan for him to get back to his own apartment and to make an immediate plan for him to get back some of the important things he lost in moving into the group home. Ed wants the following people at his meeting:*

- His primary clinical service provider. *(Ed has a supportive and trusting relationship with this provider and has asked him to facilitate the meeting.)*;
- His mother;
- His best friend, Jerome;
- And his case manager at the group home.

Exercise 2. Consider the following scenario and then discuss the questions below.
Sam's story:

> *The individual you are supporting ("Sam") has carried out a number of preplanning activities and has decided that his priority for his upcoming PCCP meeting is to discuss, and make an action plan for, his desired move from the group home to a supervised apartment setting. He has asked that you help him arrange a meeting and to invite his aunt. After Sam leaves the office, his aunt returns your phone call and explains to you how excited she is to be invited to the meeting. She is very relieved that she will be able to work with you to convince Sam that this is a terrible decision. The aunt needs orientation regarding her role in the upcoming PCCP meeting.*

1. How might you orient Sam's aunt to the PCCP process?
2. What rights of Sam's need to be respected here?
3. Think about meetings you have been involved in that have gone well, and list the reasons.
4. Think about meetings that have gone poorly and to list the reasons.

Exercise 3.

The following is a sample PCCP process observation tool that can help you to reflect on the degree to which your PCCP meetings stay true to several core person-centered values. Developed by a team of dedicated stakeholders from the Western Massachusetts Department of Mental Health, this tool, *Guidelines for Person-Centeredness in Planning Meetings* [5], prompts the recorder to collect process observations and to rate adherence to "person-centeredness" on a scale of 0 to 3, with 0 representing an absence of the value in the meeting and 3 representing a strong presence of the value in the meeting.

Ask to sit in on a peer's recovery planning meeting and complete the *Guidelines for Person-Centeredness* tool. Invite your peer to do the same for one of your upcoming planning meetings. Following the mutual observations, meet to compare the notes and discuss the following questions.

1. After filling out this questionnaire, what key areas of person-centered process do you feel are already strong in practice?
2. What key areas need the most attention? How might these areas be strengthened?
3. What were you most surprised about in completing this exercise?

Guidelines for Person-Centeredness in Planning Meetings:

A Process Observation Tool

(Davidow, S., Simms, N., Sprung, S., & Swenson, C., 2012).

1. TONE AND RELATIONSHIP:

- **Equality**. *There is a sense that everyone in the meeting is equal to everyone else, as human beings, even though they are playing different roles and have different struggles.*
- **Respect, Concern, Warmth**. *The tone includes warmth, concern, and respect.*
- **Common Language**. *Common language is used, understandable to all, free of unnecessary medical or clinical words.*
- **Full Attention**. *People pay full attention: no cell phone activity or sidebar conversations.*
- **Checking In**. *The facilitator "checks in" periodically to see if meeting is helpful; if the individual is silent, that is, accepted, and the facilitator works to involve him or her.*

3	2.5	2	1.5	1	0.5	0
STRONG		MODERATE		MINIMAL		ABSENT

• *Meeting is on time and in a comfortable space* • *Begins with introductions and orientation* • *Tone is warm and respectful* • *Individual is addressed directly* • *Facilitator works respectfully to involve the silent individual* • *Participants pay full attention—no cell phones, sidebar conversations* • *Person-first language is used (e.g., "individual diagnosed with X")* • *Common, understandable language is used—not unnecessary medical or clinical words* • *Facilitator checks in periodically to see if meeting is helpful*	• *Meeting time and space are not prompt and comfortable* • *Meeting is led in casual manner with insufficient orientation* • *Tone is disrespectful, judgmental, noncollaborative* • *Individual is talked about, rather than included or addressed* • *Participants are distracted by phones, sidebar conversations* • *Person-first language is not used (e.g., "schizophrenic")* • *Technical, medical, and clinical terms are used unnecessarily* • *Facilitator makes no effort to check in about whether meeting is helpful*

2. GOALS

- **Determination of Goals**. *Stated goals are those of the individual, and in his or her words. They articulate his or her dreams, values, and life choices. Choices of the individual are respected, even when the stated goals differ from those recommended by providers.*

- **Types of Goals**. *The goals are about having a meaningful life in the community, which may or may not include a reduction in symptoms.*
- **Unarticulated Goals**. *When the individual has not or cannot articulate his/her goals, providers assist him/her in defining them.*
- **Timeline for Accomplishment**. *The timeline for accomplishing goals will vary from person to person; it should be based on a flexible schedule to allow time to build relationships and foster trust.*

3	2.5	2	1.5	1	0.5	0
STRONG		MODERATE		MINIMAL		ABSENT

<table>
<tr>
<td>

- *Stated goals are those of the individual in his/her own words.*
- *Individual's goals are respected even if they differ from goals recommended by providers.*
- *The goals are about having a meaningful life in the community, which may or may not include a reduction in symptoms.*
- *When individual does not spell out his/her goals, providers assist him/her in defining them.*
- *Timeline for accomplishing goals is flexible, allowing time for individual to gain needed trust.*

</td>
<td>

- *Providers' goals take precedence over individual's goals, which are dismissed, ignored, or considered unrealistic.*
- *Goals are primarily about "treatment compliance," reduction of symptoms, and risk.*
- *If individual does not spell out goals, providers do little to help elicit and define them.*
- *Timelines for goal accomplishment are set arbitrarily by providers.*

</td>
</tr>
</table>

3. PROBLEM SOLVING

- **Action Steps**. *Once the individual's goals are identified, the facilitator works with the individual and other participants to specify realistic action steps.*
- **Obstacles**. *In identifying goals and action steps, the facilitator works with the individual and other participants to identify obstacles.*
- **Resources**. *The facilitator works with everyone to specify resources for accomplishing goals and overcoming obstacles.*
- **Assignments**. *Agreements are made as to who will be responsible for carrying out action steps.*

3	2.5	2	1.5	1	0.5	0
STRONG		MODERATE		MINIMAL		ABSENT

• *Facilitator works with the individual and other participants to specify action steps to goals.* • *Facilitator works with the individual and other participants to identify obstacles to goals.* • *Facilitator works with the individual and other participants to specify resources to overcome obstacles and accomplish goals.* • *Agreements are made as to who will be responsible for carrying out action steps.*	• *There is little to no effort to spell out action steps toward goals.* • *There is little to no effort to identify obstacles to goals.* • *There is little to no effort to specify resources to overcome obstacles and accomplish goals.* • *No agreements are made as to who will be responsible for various goal-directed tasks.*

4. STRENGTH-BASED

- **Assumption of Strengths**. *Everyone in the meeting assumes that the individual has a core of capabilities and talents that will be important to accomplishing goals.*
- **Identification and Validation of Strengths**. *These strengths are identified and validated, if possible, in the meeting.*
- **Building on Strengths**. *Providers partner with the individual in a way that supports the use of these strengths, talents, accomplishments, and positive qualities.*
- **Allowing Strengths to Emerge Over Time**. *If it is not possible, in the meeting, to identify and build on the individual's strengths, it is still assumed that they do exist and that they will emerge over time.*

3	2.5	2	1.5	1	0.5	0
STRONG		MODERATE		MINIMAL		ABSENT

• *Providers seek out, mention, validate, and value the individual's capabilities and talents.* • *Providers emphasize the centrality of the individual's strengths in plans to overcome obstacles and accomplish goals.* • *If the individual's strengths are not identifiable during the meeting, providers indicate that they assume the strengths will become apparent over time.*	• *Providers show little to no interest in identifying and valuing the individual's capabilities and talents, but highlight deficits, symptoms, and risk.* • *In plans to help the individual realize goals, providers emphasize "outside" resources, overlooking the individual's capabilities and talents.* • *Providers give up easily on the attempt to identify and build on the individual's strengths.*

5. SELF-DETERMINATION

- **Level of Participation**. *The individual has as active a role as he or she desires in the conduct of the meeting.*
- **Determination of Goals and Methods**. *It is understood and accepted that the individual may change his or her mind, wish to take a different path, or be more fluid in his or her goals.*
- **Leadership**. *If the individual provides leadership and direction, staff members respectfully follow that lead.*
- **Sign Off**. *Whether or not the individual provides leadership, staff members still look to him or her to sign off on the details of the plan, either during the meeting or in reviewing notes and plans later.*

3	2.5	2	1.5	1	0.5	0
STRONG		MODERATE		MINIMAL		ABSENT

• *Providers invite and support the individual taking as active a role as he or she desires in the conduct of the meeting.* • *Providers respect the leadership of the individual in defining and redefining goals and how to accomplish them.* • *If the individual provides leadership and direction, staff members respectfully follow.* • *Whether the individual provides leadership or not, providers still look to him or her to sign off on the details of the plan, during or following the meeting*	• *Providers behave as if they are, and should be, in the "driver's seat," having more expertise, wisdom, and experience than the individual.* • *There is little room or support for the individual to provide leadership.* • *There is no apparent evidence that providers will seek out the individual's sign off on the plan, in the meeting or later.* • *Providers' apparent fear of the consequences of supporting the individual's self-determination totally overrides any support for self-determination or for working toward elimination of safety-related restrictions.*

6. SENSITIVITY TO CULTURE, CONTEXT, HISTORY, AND TRAUMA

- **Language**. *Meetings are conducted in the preferred language of the individual, or an interpreter is found.*
- **Cultural and Spiritual Beliefs**. *During the course of discussion and planning, providers demonstrate awareness of and sensitivity to the individual's cultural background, cultural views, spiritual beliefs, and interest in alternative healing practices.*
- **Trauma-Informed**. *Similarly, in the meeting and in the process of planning, providers are sensitive to the effects of abuse and trauma, including awareness of the trauma that results from episodes of illness and treatment. Providers collaborate with the individual to find a suitable approach to the discussion of trauma.*

3	2.5	2	1.5	1	0.5	0
STRONG		MODERATE		MINIMAL		ABSENT

- *The meeting is conducted in the individual's preferred language or an interpreter is found.*
- *Providers show awareness of, interest in, and sensitivity to, the individual's cultural background and views, spiritual beliefs, and interest in alternative healing practices, which are incorporated into the plan when the individual so desires.*
- *Providers show awareness of, interest in, and sensitivity to, the effects of abuse and trauma on the individual, including the trauma of some episodes of illness and treatment, and apply these insights in treatment planning.*
- *Providers collaborate with the individual to find a suitable approach to the discussion of trauma.*

- *The meeting is not conducted in the individual's preferred language, and no effort was made to find an interpreter.*
- *There is evidence that providers not only do not mention, appreciate, or highlight cultural, historical, familial, or trauma-related factors, but also actively block inclusion of these crucial factors in the conversation or in treatment planning.*

7. COMMUNITY RESOURCES

- **Prioritizing Community Resources**. *Providers demonstrate an interest in and priority on locating community resources (outside the mental health system) relevant to the individual's goals and desires.*
- **Accessing Community Resources**. *If the individual desires, providers offer support in accessing and connecting with those resources (e.g., classes, groups, activities, programs, churches).*
- **Accessing Self-Help Resources**. *If the individual desires, effort is put into identifying, locating, and accessing local self-help resources.*

3	2.5	2	1.5	1	0.5	0
STRONG		MODERATE		MINIMAL		ABSENT

• Providers show an interest in helping the individual locate community resources (outside the mental health system) relevant to his or her goals and desires. • If the individual desires, providers offer support in accessing and connecting with those resources (e.g., classes, groups, activities, programs, churches). • If the individual desires, effort is put into identifying, locating, and accessing local self-help resources.	• Providers show little interest in identifying local community resources for the person outside the mental health system, and even appear to actively discourage it. • Statements are made that for purposes of safety, the person should just connect with resources and programs within the mental health system. • Providers evidence no interest in helping the individual locate and use local self-help resources.

8. WISDOM OF RISK

- **Supporting Risk.** *Providers support the individual in taking risks as part of growing and learning.*
- **Learning from Risk Taking.** *If the individual has recently taken risks that led to unsafe outcomes or negative consequences, providers highlight the opportunity to learn rather than highlighting the failure.*

3	2.5	2	1.5	1	0.5	0
STRONG		MODERATE		MINIMAL		ABSENT

• Providers reinforce efforts and statements by the individual in taking risks in the service of growth and learning, even if they are worried about the outcomes. • If concerned about risks the individual is taking, providers try to engage him or her in a balanced dialogue about possible unsafe outcomes and ways to minimize those. • If the individual has recently taken risks that led to unsafe or negative consequences, providers highlight the opportunity to learn from the incidents rather than highlighting the failure.	• Providers clearly discourage risk-taking behaviors, equating them with negative outcomes and danger. • Providers fail to engage the individual in a balanced dialogue that respects the wisdom of risk and at the same time the potential for unsafe outcomes. • In response to recent risk taking by the individual that led to unsafe outcomes, providers highlight the failure and the need for compliance in the future, without encouraging a discussion of learning from the incident(s).

9. ADDRESSING SAFETY CONCERNS

- **Open Discussions About Safety**. *Providers engage the individual in a balanced dialogue about activities that could lead to unsafe outcomes, during which the individual's self-determination is respected.*
- **Determining What Is Unsafe**. *As the individual and providers may differ in identifying what is "unsafe," advocates for the individual may be included in determining safety concerns.*
- **Partnering to Promote Safety**. *If the individual and providers agree about certain behaviors posing a risk to safety, providers partner with the individual in deciding how to promote safety.*
- **Eliciting Individual's Preferences**. *If the individual and providers do not agree about certain behaviors posing a risk to safety, providers try to elicit the preferences of the individual about the handling of those provider concerns.*
- **Using Advanced Directives**. *The provider partners with the individual to support his or her use of advanced directives such as a Wellness Recovery Action Plan (WRAP) or relapse prevention tools.*

3	2.5	2	1.5	1	0.5	0
STRONG		MODERATE		MINIMAL		ABSENT

- *The individual is invited to partner with providers in determining whether certain behaviors pose safety concerns.*
- *If the individual and the providers differ in identifying what is "unsafe," the individual's views are respected, and providers suggest that an advocate for the individual be identified to join in the discussion.*
- *When providers and the individual agree about certain behaviors being unsafe, providers partner with the individual in determining how to minimize unsafe consequences.*
- *When providers and the individual do not agree about what is unsafe, providers try to elicit the individual's preferences regarding the future handling of provider concerns.*
- *The provider partners with the individual to support the use of advanced directives such as a WRAP or relapse prevention tools.*

- *There is evidence that the provider has little tolerance for trying to engage with the individual around safety concerns, preferring to move rather quickly to take control of the situation even if it means sacrificing the individual's autonomy, dignity, and willingness to collaborate.*

10. USING PEER-BASED SERVICES AND SUPPORTS

- **Accessing Peer Support Services**. *Information regarding the role and availability of peer support services is ready prior to the meeting.*
- **Deciding Whether to Use Peer Supports**. *The individual has an opportunity to meet with peer support workers or any other advocates ahead of time to determine whether their participation would be useful and whether he or she would like to invite them to the meeting.*
- **Choosing One's Own Advocates**. *The individual is invited to bring any person to the meeting as an advocate; this person may or may not be a peer worker, and may or may not be associated with that provider organization.*
- **Respect for Peer Support Workers**. *Peer support workers and other advocates are as highly regarded as any other meeting participant.*

3		2.5		2		1.5		1		0.5		0
STRONG				MODERATE				MINIMAL				ABSENT

- *The individual is informed of the availability of peer support services prior to the meeting.*
- *The individual has the opportunity to meet with any peer support worker before the meeting, and then to decide whether to invite that person to the meeting.*
- *The individual is invited to bring any person to the meeting as an advocate, whether or not the person is a peer support worker.*
- *Peer support workers and other advocates are treated as highly regarded meeting participants.*

- *Providers pay no attention to the availability or use of peer support services for the individual.*
- *Providers actually appear to be discouraging of the use of peer-based services, either seeing them as irrelevant to the overall treatment or expecting them to do more harm than good.*

11. CIRCLE OF SUPPORT

- **Invitation List**. *The provider partners with the individual in advance of the meeting to make up an invitation list; this includes providers, advocates, family members, friends, and anyone else the individual would find to be a support.*
- **The Right to Un-invite Anyone**. *If there are people who the individual would prefer not to have in the meeting, they will not be invited.*
- **Respect for the Circle of Support**. *The provider is welcoming to people in the meeting who are part of the individual's circle of support, and creates space for all guests to participate.*

3	2.5	2	1.5	1	0.5	0
STRONG		MODERATE		MINIMAL		ABSENT

- *The provider partners with the individual in advance of the meeting to make up an invitation list, to include providers, advocates, family members, friends, and anyone else the individual would like to invite.*
- *If there are people who the individual would prefer not to have in the meeting, they will not be invited.*
- *The provider is welcoming to people in the meeting who are part of the individual's circle of support, and creates space for all guests to participate.*

- *Providers show little to no interest in encouraging the individual to contribute to make an invitation list.*
- *In fact, there is evidence, explicitly or more subtly, that the provider(s) actually discourages the person served from bringing supportive individuals to a planning meeting; the provider seems to prefer not to have them.*
- *The individual is given no support to the "uninvited" or excludes certain people from the meeting.*
- *If the individual has brought a "circle of support" to the meeting, the providers do not encourage their participation.*

Learning Assessment

Module 5: Creating the Plan through a Team Meeting		
Statement	True	False
1. It is necessary for individuals to attain clinical stability prior to pursuing recovery goals such as employment.		
2. Interventions should avoid duplicating accessible supports found naturally in the community.		
3. Persuasion may be an essential skill for the PCCP facilitator.		
4. Individuals are encouraged to take on a leadership role in the PCCP process.		
5. People cannot be members of the PCCP team if they cannot attend the planning meeting.		
See the Answer Key at the end of the chapter for the correct answers. **Number Correct**		
0 to 2: You have a lot to learn. We hope you find this guide useful in the process! 3 to 4: You have a solid foundation. Use this guide to enhance your skills. 5: You are ahead of the game! Use this guide to teach others and strive for **excellence!**		

References

1. Mount R, Riggs D, Brown M, Hibbard M. (2003) *Moving On: A Personal Futures Planning Workbook for Individuals with Brain Injury*, 2nd Edition. Research and Training Center on Community Integration of Individuals with TBI, Mount Sinai Medical Center, New York, NY.
2. Tondora J, Pocklington S, Gregory GA *et al.* (2005). *Implementation of Person-Centered Care and Planning: How Philosophy can Inform Practice.* Substance Abuse and Mental Health Services Administration, Rockville, MD.
3. California Department of Education. (2002) *Direct Support Professional Training Resource Guide: Communication, Problem-Solving and Conflict Resolution.* Department of Education and the Regional Occupational Centers and Program in partnership with the Department of Developmental Services, CA.
4. Mead S, Copeland ME. (2000) What recovery means to us: Consumers' perspectives. *Community Mental Health Journal* **36**, 315-328.
5. Davidow, S, Simms, N, Sprung, S, Swenson, C, (2012). *Guidelines for Person-Centeredness in Recovery Planning Meetings: A Process Observation Tool.* Western Massachusetts, Department of Mental Health.

Answers to the Learning Assessment:

1. F
2. T
3. T
4. T
5. F

Module 6: Documentation of PCCP: Writing the plan to honor the person AND satisfy the chart

Goal

This module details how to reflect person-centered principles and practices in the documentation of the written recovery plan. Strategies are presented for maximizing the recovery orientation of the plan and meeting the rigorous documentation expectations of fiscal and accrediting bodies.

Learning Objectives

After completing this module, you will be better able to:

- define the key documentation components (i.e., goals, objectives, and interventions) of the person-centered care planning (PCCP) as a roadmap to recovery and wellness;
- note two ways in which PCCP documentation differs from the traditional written treatment plans;
- write meaningful short-term objectives that reflect the S-M-A-R-T criteria;
- create and record rigorous person-centered care plans that support the individual's recovery while meeting regulatory and payer requirements.

Learning Assessment

A learning assessment is included at the end of the module. If you are already familiar with this subject, you may want to go to the end of this module and take the assessment to see how much you know already. Then you can focus your learning efforts on what is new for you.

Partnering for Recovery in Mental Health: A Practical Guide to Person-Centered Planning, First Edition. Janis Tondora, Rebecca Miller, Mike Slade and Larry Davidson. © 2014 John Wiley & Sons, Ltd. Published 2014 by John Wiley & Sons, Ltd.

Introduction to the Documentation of Person-Centered Care Plans

As previously stated, person-centered care planning (PCCP) consists of four components: philosophy, process, plan, and product. We have previously discussed philosophy and process, and this module focuses on this third "P" of documenting the *written care plan*. Specifically, we address a question that is frequently posed by practitioners working on PCCP: *Is it possible to write a plan that honors the person while still satisfying the chart, my supervisor, our funders, and so on?* This documentation section is included in recognition of the fact that many highly skilled practitioners embrace both the philosophy and the process of PCCP and yet struggle to reflect this in the context of the written planning document. Frequently, it is in this step of moving from "process" to "plan" that the quality of PCCP breaks down and the written document devolves into one that is both deficit-oriented and professionally driven rather than staying true to the principles of PCCP.

But, first, you might be wondering: "Does it really matter? The written plan is NOT something that is a meaningful part of the work … In fact, it gets in the way of the work!" If this is on your mind, you have lots of company! Frequently, the written plan is viewed simply as a technical document that has to be completed to satisfy accrediting or reimbursement bodies, and is seen as useful neither to the practitioner nor to the person receiving care. In such cases, the plan is completed and filed in the medical record and it plays a little, if any, role in actually guiding the work of the team moving forward. While this may be a widely held perception of care planning documentation, in the person-centered world, the plan of care has the potential and should be far more than a paperwork requirement. It is a written contract between a person and his or her network of supporters that outlines a more hopeful vision for the future and how all will work together to achieve it. The pivotal role of the service plan in transforming systems of mental health care was perhaps best described in the US President's New Freedom Commission Report [1], which noted that customized plans should be developed in full partnership with consumers as "the plan of care is at the core of the consumer-centered, recovery oriented system."

> The plan of care has the potential, and should be, far more than a paperwork requirement …

Given the centrality of the PCCP in driving system change, it is imperative that practitioners increase their competency in creating collaboratively developed documents that "honor the person while also satisfying the chart." But for many practitioners, developing these skills may take practice if they differ significantly from their typical style of care planning documentation. This section is therefore intended to support practitioners in the *practical* implementation of PCCP by presenting a general overview of the core documentation elements along with tips for maximizing the person-centered aspects of each. It is not intended to substitute for the rich discussion of philosophy and process that has preceded this module, as the quality of the planning document is only as good as the values and partnership on which it is based. Put simply, all four "Ps" need to come together for the vision of PCCP to become a reality. In addition, this module is not intended to be a "compliance" guide for meeting specific care planning documentation requirements. These requirements vary widely across states, counties, and particular programs, and, as such, a discussion of these is beyond the scope of this module. Here we focus more on the larger question of "quality" rather than the specific requirements of "compliance."

Medical Necessity and Documentation of the PCCP

Medical necessity refers to the expectation that services are provided to impact a diagnosed condition that is causing symptoms, distress, and/or functional impairment, and that is likely to improve as a result of the proposed treatment or intervention. Typically, services are paid for under an insurance plan only if they meet the criteria for medical necessity. In many settings, medical necessity also establishes a standard of service and quality of care. One aspect of quality care is about doing the right thing, at the right time, for the right reason. While a care plan can include many options (including action steps taken by the person in recovery as well as any natural supporters who may be involved), practitioners will be paid by insurance programs only for those services that meet medical necessity criteria, that is, the rationale for providing the service is clear as it relates to helping the person to overcome clearly documented mental health-related impairments that are negatively impacting his or her life and functioning. It is important to note that the interventions do not have to reduce or eliminate the condition altogether to be considered medically necessary. Rather, interventions may be considered necessary if they are required by the nature of the person's condition in order for him or her to be able to live the meaningful and dignified life of his or her choice.

Because of this required link back to mental health symptoms or impairments, many practitioners believe that the construct of "medical necessity" is wholly incompatible with the goal-oriented, strength-based nature of person-centered care plans. Some have described it as feeling "caught between a rock and a hard place." On the one hand, they must write a plan that honors the person's valued goals, strengths, and priorities. On the other hand, that same plan needs to meet a whole host of external requirements set forth by regulatory bodies and funders.

It is the reality of the current mental health system that the requirements of primary payers such as Medicare and Medicaid are difficult to balance in the context of creating person-centered care plans. However, practitioners are encouraged to learn about their state's Medicaid plan(s) in detail prior to making an assumption that meeting medical necessity criteria is an insurmountable challenge. More information and understanding of the real and perceived barriers to doing PCCP is needed, as there have been developments in recent years that have widened the scope of reimbursable services (such as those provided under the Rehabilitation Option) and established new funding mechanisms (such as self-directed budgeting pilots).

In addition, contrary to common myths in the field, the documentation of PCCP need not be "soft" in any way. In fact, emerging practice guidelines explicitly call for the documentation of (i) comprehensive clinical formulations, (ii) mental health-related barriers that interfere with functioning, (iii) strengths and resources, (iv) short-term, measurable objectives, and (v) clearly articulated interventions that spell out who is doing what on which timeline and for what purpose [2, 3]. We suggest that these standards for PCCP documentation are on par with, if not superior to, the level of rigor that actually exists in most clinical and rehabilitation plans around the country, and believe that the documentation tips provided below support, rather than undermine, compliance with regulatory requirements. Medical necessity and person-centered care are not incompatible constructs, and service plans can be created in partnership with persons in recovery while also maintaining rigorous standards around treatment and documentation.

While plans can be quite elaborate and detailed, a person-centered care plan contains several core elements that are depicted in Figure 6.1 and described in greater detail in this module.

Many people find that the terms presented in Figure 6.1 are not entirely intuitive and have difficulty in differentiating each of the elements. It is important that early on, in learning about PCCP, there is a clear understanding of these essential, and distinct, documentation components.

Goals

The creation of the PCCP document should flow from goal statements that reflect what the person receiving services would like to achieve in his or her life. Goals are decided following a thorough strength-based assessment as described in Module 4 and through a collaborative

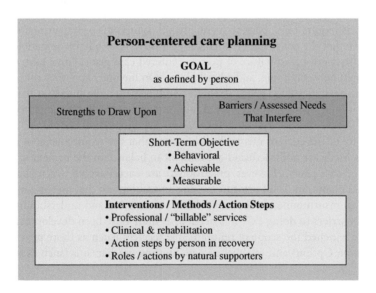

Figure 6.1   Core Elements in a Person-Centered Care Plan

dialogue (see Module 5) with the person receiving services and his or her team. The key elements of goal(s) within a person-centered care plan are described below:

Goals: Important to the Person

> A well-written goal statement on a PCCP reflects that which is important to the focus person rather than that which historically has been given priority in the professional service system.

Ideally, the goal is expressed in the person's own words and is based on his or her unique interests, preferences, and strengths. A goal is a statement of something important for an individual to achieve in his or her personal recovery. It may be a life goal, a treatment goal, or a goal to improve the quality of the person's life. This approach to a goal statement can be quite different from the manner

> *If of thy mortal goods thou art bereft,*
> *And from thy slender store*
> *Two loaves alone to thee are left,*
> *Sell one, and with the dole*
> *Buy hyacinths to feed thy soul.*
>
> -- *Sa'adi* [4]

in which goals are typically documented in professionally driven service plans. Traditionally, goals are focused more narrowly on the amelioration of symptoms or deficits associated with the mental health condition (e.g., behaviors, functional limitations) thereby losing the focus on personally valued and meaningful life goals. Goals, for example, to remain medication compliant, reduce behavioral outbursts, maintain stability, and increase insight are commonly listed on service plans despite the fact that persons in recovery rarely see these things as meaningful or motivating long-term outcomes. This is not to say that these things are necessarily negative or undesirable. But, reducing symptoms, increasing compliance, and staying out of the hospital are *means to an end* and they do not, in and of themselves, equate with the realization of a person's ultimate vision for his or her future.

Therefore, in supporting individuals to either develop or modify their PCCP goals, it is important for practitioners to keep in mind that the goals of the plan should not be limited to clinically valued or professionally determined outcomes. Rather, goals should be defined by the person with a focus on attaining the life he or she envisions for himself or herself in the community. A well-written goal statement on a PCCP reflects that which is important to the focus person rather than that which historically has been given priority in the professional service system.

> *"How would your life look different if [this problem] were gone?"*

Ideally, such goals are written in *positive* language, remembering that this is an opportunity to embody and reinforce hope and growth. A goal is best thought of as something to move toward rather than something to get rid of. For example, in working with individuals to identify a recovery goal for their care plan, it is not uncommon for people to stick to the territory they are most accustomed to exploring with treatment teams. You may hear, "I just want to be less depressed," or even, "I want the voices to quiet down." Rather than accepting this as the final goal for the plan, a skilled practitioner will go deeper and ask the individual, "If you were less depressed, or if the voices were quiet, can you tell me how your life would be different? What would you be doing every day? What kinds of things might you enjoy? What would be different?" Most often, this type of inquiry in the goal-setting process will generate PCCP goal statements that focus on the following types of areas:

Managing own life - *I want to control my own money.*
Work/education - *I want to finish school.*
Spiritual issues - *I want to get back to church.*
Satisfying relationships - *I want to see my grandkids.*
Adequate housing - *I want to move out of the group home.*
Social activities - *I want to join a bowling league.*
Health/well-being - *I want to lose weight.*

Goals: A Manageable Number

Sometimes people articulate multiple goals, sometimes none at all. Each scenario presents different challenges.

Too many goals?

In this case, it is most effective to help the person to prioritize and identify just a few key goal areas on the plan. Having too many goals can make the plan complicated and unwieldy—both for the practitioner to write and, most importantly, for the person to actually "work" out that plan in his or her daily life! In order for the plan to be a truly effective tool in guiding recovery, it is helpful to limit the goal statements to those that are most salient and motivating to the individual at that point in time. Often, the most powerful and effective plans are focused only on one larger goal. This does not mean that the person does not have goals or challenges in other areas that might ultimately need to be addressed, but it can be helpful to give dedicated attention to a specific area over a defined time frame while deferring other goals to a future plan.

An important reminder: As discussed in Module 4, take care in the goal-setting and prioritization process; do not "table" what is most *important to* the person, including only that which you think is *important for* them from a clinical or professional perspective.

No goals?

How about the alternative scenario? Practitioners often ask: *What do I do if the person has NO goals or if he or she is content with the way things are?* First, remember that most people do not live their lives explicitly in terms of "goals," and the person may not be accustomed to being asked about life goals beyond those usually identified in treatment. Previous experiences of care planning may have involved limited participation; perhaps the person was only expected to lend a signature after the written document had been created. This highlights the shift in roles and responsibilities that occurs in PCCP, and underscores the importance of the preplanning steps detailed in Module 2. If PCCP is about getting the person in the "driver's seat" to the maximum extent possible, then some people will benefit from "driver's education" so they can be fully prepared to partner with their team from start to finish.

The practitioner and other team members, including peer specialists, play an important role in this process by maintaining a positive attitude and focusing on the possibilities for the future rather than the challenges. Put simply, practitioners may need to be "holders of hope" in situations in which the focus person is having difficulty expressing goals or a more positive vision for the future. A spirit of hope is communicated in attitude as well as through the specific tools she or he uses throughout the PCCP process. For example, it is essential that practitioners be skilled in the use of strength-based assessment and motivational enhancement techniques as these can be particularly helpful in supporting individuals to rediscover (or discover for the first time!) goals and dreams that they may have lost along the way.

In this way, being person-centered does not mean refraining from offering suggestions or ideas when a person is stuck about what they would like to work on. Ideas may emerge at any time during conversations or sessions, and these might be revisited around the time of planning. Here is an example: one of us, while assisting in preparing a plan with some-one receiving services, asked: "Do you have any goals you'd like to work on?" and received a resounding and desultory "no" for the answer. Yet when asked if the person was interested in working, the person answered in the affirmative and offered several job ideas. Entering into the conversation from a "side door" rather than head-on can be helpful, as can sugges-tions and reminders of previously mentioned interests and goals from prior conversations. Important to stress, though, is continuing to utilize strong clinical skills and judgment in determining whether a friendly suggestion is being taken instead as a command or dictum. Awareness of power and authority is essential in the PCCP goal setting process just as it is in any productive therapeutic practice or relationship.

Goals: Time Framed?

Goals may be set for a shorter or longer period of time. Depending on the funder require-ments and the regulations of your state and agency, time frames for goal statements may, or may not, need to be specified on the recovery plan. The important thing to remember is that the scope of goal statements should vary depending on an individual's personal preferences and current priorities. The goal may be 5 years down the road, or something that may be accomplished in the next 6 months. For example, a person may prefer, and be highly moti-vated, to set an ambitious long-term goal such as "Graduating from college," which may take several years to accomplish. Another individual may feel overwhelmed at the scope of such a task, and might prefer to start with a goal of "Completing a class at the local Adult Education Department," which may be achieved within a much shorter period of time.

Goals: Attainable and Realistic?

Ideally, the identified goal is attainable and realistic for the individual—but there may be times when there is disagreement on this issue. Whether or not a practitioner views a given person's goal as feasible need not become a source of conflict or disagreement or a barrier to developing the plan. For example, if a practitioner is concerned that a person's stated goal is unrealistic, this goal might be preserved out of respect for the individual's preferences and understanding of his or her own recovery. Practitioners cannot predict the future, and should not presume to do so. In fact, many people currently working as peer staff within the mental health system report being told by practitioners earlier in their recovery that they would never be able to return to work because of the severity of their illness. Such pronouncements are not only demoralizing, but also convey a sense of certainty that is simply not warranted by the available data.

When crafting the goal statements for the service plan, it is far more helpful for the practitioner to help the person to THINK BIG as this is an opportunity to demonstrate faith and hope in their recovery process. A word of caution NOT to become overly concerned with whether or not the goal statement is "realistic" as determining what is realistic (or not) is a slippery slope and often allows unspoken biases or assumptions to come into play. There will be places later in the care planning document (most notably the short-term objectives discussed later in this module) to carve out smaller "achievable" first steps but, for the purpose of the goal statement, it is most helpful to retain the long-term goal that is most motivating for the individual. During the initial goal-setting process, the practitioner and/or peer specialist should therefore remind all team members to refrain from making comments that reflect skepticism or doubt regarding the feasibility of the long-term recovery vision.

There are times when the practitioner will have a different sense of priority goals and is often inclined—by virtue of training, experience, and even at times legal obligations or mandates. In most cases, practitioners view basic health and safety needs for food, clothing, shelter, and medical care, if indicated, as a first priority. On the other hand, a not uncommon point of difference is when co-occurring drug or alcohol use confounds the picture. In these circumstances, a harm reduction strategy might be a reasonable approach. Regardless, some recognition of the differences and negotiation to a point of shared priorities is essential if the rest of the PCCP process is to succeed. Consider the following example.

A man who was receiving services in a mental health program had the misfortune of having three different mental health providers in one year. The first provider met with the man to do a treatment plan with him. The provider asked the man: "What are your goals?" The man responded: "Well, I really want to be an astronaut!" The provider attributed the statement to the man's ongoing delusions; believed that other things were a bigger priority; and was concerned that to allow such a goal would be "setting him up" for failure. The provider suggested he needed to focus on finding a new place to live because his lease was up. "First things first," he said as he wrote the housing goal in the plan. Even after the man had secured an apartment, there was no further follow-up about the man's interest in becoming an astronaut.

Six months later, it was time for the man's review and he met a new provider. This provider sat with the man, looked over the plan, and asked: "What are your goals?" Once again, the man responded: "I really want to be an astronaut!!" The provider, who made little eye contact with the man while he wrote furiously on the document, responded that he had been to the man's apartment and felt that he really needed to work on his ADL (activities of daily living) skills. The provider wrote this on the review, and tabled the man's goal of being an astronaut as unrealistic – a grandiose idea that did not warrant further exploration.

Six months later ... new review ... new provider. By this time, the man had just about given up. The new provider sat down with the man and asked him: "What are your goals?" The man, knowing what he really wanted, responded: "I REALLY want to be an astronaut!!!" This provider looked directly at the man and said: "Okay, here's the deal. Go to the library. Get all of the information you can about what you will need to do to be an astronaut and I will do some research too. Bring the information back in two weeks and we'll discuss it together." The man left encouraged for the first time in a long time.

Two weeks later, the man came back and plopped a sheaf of papers on the desk of the provider and declared: "I can't possibly do all of this! I need to have a Ph.D. in physics, be an officer in the military, go through all of these tests and physicals ... this is too much!" The provider smiled inwardly, but did not blink an eye as he said: "Okay, don't give up yet. What were the things about being an astronaut that most appealed to you? What about it gets you excited?" Over the next several sessions, they worked on the things that the man could do to realize certain parts of the dream.

Fortunately, the man and his provider were located in Houston, Texas, very close to the Kennedy Space Center. The provider helped the man to meet people in different capacities there and eventually the man did get a job. While working, the man met a pilot who gave skydiving lessons on the weekends. He tried it and loved it. In skydiving, the man found much of the same freedom and adventure he had sought in his dream of being an astronaut.

Story provided by Sade Ali, Advisory Board Member,
SAMHSA Person-Directed Planning Initiative

This story illustrates the importance of "listening" to and understanding people's priorities as you work together to establish goals for the person-centered plan. Imagine the impact on the helping relationship when this man was repeatedly dismissed and told that his dream of becoming an astronaut needed to take a backseat to the goals that each of his providers deemed important. While it is true that providers often have an obligation to help ensure that an individual's basic needs (e.g., housing) or clinical needs (e.g., acute symptoms) are addressed, it is essential to balance this with a simultaneous appreciation for needs and goals as expressed by the person. Doing so can lead the individual to discover a whole range of new experiences that serve to further his or her own personal recovery process.

Goals: Something We Get Paid For?

Goals discovered through the PCCP process frequently will involve the types of statements noted earlier in this module, that is, *I want to go back to church … have a girlfriend … join a bowling league,* and so on. Practitioners and administrators have expressed concern that these written goal statements will not be allowed by internal or external compliance and regulatory bodies, as they are not consistent with their mission to provide a particular professional service, for example, *We are in the mental health business and these goals don't sound very "mental-health-like!"* This belief that funders will not pay for nonclinical life goals is actually a correct one, but not because of the nature of the goal itself. Rather, it is the fact that *funders do not pay for goals at all.* Funders pay practitioners for the *interventions and other professional services* they provide to help people overcome mental health-related *barriers* that interfere with their functioning and attainment of valued personal goals. So, for the many PCCP practitioners who, by necessity, must also concern themselves with regulatory compliance and "medical necessity," keep in mind that there *will* be places within your plan documentation for you to build this "business case." However, more so than any other part of the plan, the goal statement truly belongs to the individual and it should honor his or her unique vision for the future.

Goals: A Note on the Stage of Change

It is important to remember that goal statements on a PCCP may look very different depending on a person's readiness to change and level of engagement in services. Goals focusing on life changes presume a preparatory or action stage of change as well as a belief on the part of the person that mental health services can help him/her to make such a desired change. Some people may still be in the process developing a trusting and working relationship with the practitioner and service agency, so they may have difficulty engaging in active goal setting. The goal in such cases might simply be engagement, and may be something first identified by the practitioner. The goal may also be identified as something like "I want to get mental health practitioners and treatment out of my life," for those who want to stop receiving services. Even in such cases, developing collaborative goals is often the first step toward building the trust needed for the person to give treatment a chance to make a positive difference in his or her life.

Strengths and Barriers

Once the goal has been identified, the next step in creating a plan is to identify those specific strengths that will support the person in attaining the goal, and those barriers (including mental health and addiction-related barriers) that stand in the way of goal achievement.

Strengths

Focusing solely on deficits and barriers in the absence of a thoughtful analysis of strengths disregards the most critical resources an individual has on which to build in his or her efforts to achieve life goals and dreams. Thus, it is considered a key practice in PCCP to thoughtfully consider the potential strengths and resources of the focus person as well as his or her family, natural support network, and community at large. For this reason, a key role of the practitioner (as discussed in greater detail in Module 4) is to support the individual in identifying a diverse range of strengths, interests, and talents while also considering how to *actively use these strengths* to pursue goals and objectives in the person-centered care plan. Put simply, all too often strengths are identified in the assessment and preplanning process and yet appear nowhere on the final written document! Strengths are not identified just to "sit on a shelf."

Rather, the team needs to think creatively about how to explicitly incorporate them in the various activities within the PCCP. For example, if the focus person identifies his or her faith and spirituality as a cornerstone of well-being, are these types of activities reflected in his or her daily personal wellness plan? If the individual has a love of creative writing, is this identified as a positive coping strategy the person can use to manage stress or difficult emotions? If the person is an accomplished musician, might he or she work toward volunteering to teach music lessons to others at the local community or senior center?

This emphasis on individual and/or family "strengths" rather than deficits or problems is sometimes a difficult process for professional service practitioners as well as the service user himself or herself! It is not uncommon, for example, for individuals to have difficulty identifying their "strengths," as this has not historically been the focus of professional services and assessments. Individuals also may have lost sight of their gifts and talents through years of struggles with their disability and discrimination. As a result, simply asking the question "What are your strengths?" is seldom enough to solicit information regarding resources and capabilities that can be built on in the planning process. Guiding principles and sample questions to be used in strength-based interviewing are provided previously within this document (see Module 4 for a broader discussion and ideas for specific questions in this area).

Barriers

While capitalizing on a person's strengths, it is also necessary for the "roadblocks" that interfere with goal attainment—often in the shape of disability-related limitations, experiences, or symptoms—to be identified and addressed in the PCCP. Barriers should be acknowledged alongside assets and strengths, as this is essential not only for the purpose of justifying care and the "medical necessity" of the professional services and supports provided, but because a clear understanding of what is getting in the way informs choices of the various professional interventions and natural supports that might then be offered to the individual in the service of his or her recovery. The difference in a person-centered care plan is that the barriers do not become the *exclusive and dominant* focus of the plan and only take on meaning to the extent that they are interfering with the attainment of larger life goals. For example, the reduction of symptoms is not seen as the only desired outcome (unless the person himself or herself so chooses), but rather is noted as a way of addressing a barrier (in this case, the barrier being symptoms) in order to help the person return to work, finish school, be a better parent, pursue a hobby, and so on.

In identifying barriers, it is important to be specific. For example, at the individual level, the following types of factors might impede goal attainment:

- Intrusive or burdensome symptoms
- Lack of resources
- Need for assistance/supports
- Problems in behavior
- Need for skills development
- Challenges in taking care of oneself and activities of daily living
- Threats to basic health and safety

An Example: The individual's goal is to someday work with children, preferably in a preschool environment. However, cognitive and social impairments resulting from the effects of a mental health condition have made it difficult for the person to achieve a high school diploma (which is required for most positions in preschool education). A traditional service plan might note that the *goal* is to "reduce symptoms," "increase concentration," or perhaps "decrease paranoia."

In a PCCP, the goal is stated simply in the person's own words

I want to get my degree in education and someday be a teacher.

with perhaps a shorter term objective being to receive a GED. The following might then be noted in the barriers section of the plan:

Barriers: difficulty concentrating due to depression; previously unable to meet attendance requirements at GED class due to lack of energy and high anxiety; difficulty remembering, tracking, and completing assignments; at times uncomfortable around and fearful of other students; anxiety related to taking bus to GED classes.

These specific barriers provide targets for interventions to address and justify services through establishing the medical necessity of care.

In addition to exploring these individual-level barriers, it is important to note the extent to which *external* barriers might also be interfering with goal attainment. For example, many individuals who wish to pursue their education have difficulty securing financial aid, transportation, childcare, or classroom accommodations. A key role of the practitioner is to work with the individual and team to identify both internal and environmental barriers and to determine strategies and solutions that help the person to move forward through, under, over, or around these barriers.

Objectives

Goal statements are useful as they give direction for the overall recovery journey and all that it entails. Just as in pursuing any goal, it is essential to identify specific, shorter term action steps that can help the person to move toward his or her life goals and dreams. These steps are usually referred to as *objectives* and are best thought of as interim goals that break down longer term aspirations into meaningful and positive short-term changes. For example, in the vignette described, getting a GED was a target objective en route to a longer term goal of working with children.

A strong objective should reflect a concrete *change in functioning, in behavior, or in status*, that, when achieved, will provide the "proof" that the person is making progress. As much as possible, objectives should describe the development of *new* skills and abilities, including the ability to access the needed supports and accommodations. For instance, an individual may need to develop an ability to negotiate certain workplace accommodations from his or her employer. This kind of focus on skill building and enhancing self-management goes a long way toward promoting recovery and the person's vision of the future.

As with all parts of the written PCCP, these objectives should be arrived at only after a thoughtful dialogue with the person about what he or she feels would be a meaningful "step in the right direction." Practitioners may need to help the individual establish objectives. If the person could do it himself or herself, then he or she most likely wouldn't be seeking services! Here is where the practitioner's role as coach, collaborator, and so on is prominent. In addition to assisting the person in identifying feasible and meaningful objectives, the practitioner can then be instrumental in identifying, describing, and eventually offering the services and supports that will be useful to the person as he or she pursues his or her goals.

Objectives: How Ambitious or Modest?

The development of objectives is an area in which the practitioner can make perhaps the most significant contribution toward the person's recovery. Objectives should be defined as "doable" so that the person can move along toward a stated goal and build on incremental successes. Note that sometimes, the individual needs to try new behaviors that not everyone on the team thinks are "attainable" or "realistic." If attempting these new activities remains the person's preference, though, then the team should support that decision. The person may then succeed despite the team's concerns, or, if it is the case that the person does NOT meet the objective, the lessons learned may be productive and helpful to both the service user and practitioners. This should not be taken as a "failure" but rather an opportunity for the team to reevaluate the plan for possible modification of the objective or even the addition of a new service or support.

When service users are besieged by their problems and see little more than barriers to their goals, the discussion of short-term objectives allows the practitioner to use his or her problem solving skills to build on the individual's strengths and identify a modest and manageable step that will help move the person forward. Building on the example above, that is, a valued goal to finish school and work with children, let's assume that a major depression with psychotic features has led to multiple recent hospitalizations, and severe sleep disturbance with the individual sleeping nearly 18 hours a day. The service user may feel overwhelmed in identifying the next steps and this may prevent him/her from taking action, particularly around something as ambitious as completing the GED. This is where we see the benefit of crafting highly individualized objectives that can preserve the valued goal while truly meeting the individual where he or she is at. The individual might start with a simple

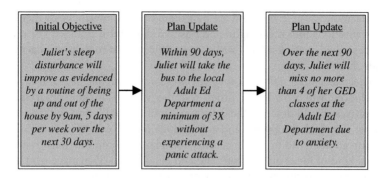

Figure 6.2   Sample of a Progressive Objective

and modest objective *to overcome her sleep disturbance as evidenced by her ability to reestablish a morning routine and be up and out of the house by 9AM, 5 days per week over the next 30 days.* Assuming the service user agrees that this would feel like a good place for her to start, such an objective moves her closer to her goal of returning to school while also clearly targeting improvement in a mental health barrier (thereby maintaining the link between the assessment and the plan and supporting medical necessity). At the same time, objectives should not be broken down to the point where they become trivial or are seen as condescending by the person served, for example, a man with a Masters Degree in Nursing who is asked to work on an objective to "verbally identify 3 negative health consequences of current diet within 6 months." Such objectives, while technically correct and easy to write, can reflect a lack of understanding of the person and his true barriers to a healthier lifestyle.

When deciding how ambitious or modest to be in setting the short-term objective, it can be helpful to remember that "progressive" objectives may be written in a sequential manner (as illustrated in Figure 6.2), that is, the achievement of one objective may trigger the activation of another in a future plan update. In this way, by dividing larger goals into smaller actions and benchmarks, objectives can provide hope to both the individual and his or her team by taking what can feel like an overwhelming journey and organizing it in a number of steps in which progress can be made and success celebrated.

Objectives: How Can I Meet All the Technical Criteria?

The writing of objectives (and interventions, to be discussed in the next section) is the most technical part of the entire PCCP documentation process, as these plan elements are closely monitored by funders and accrediting bodies. Supporting individuals to make progress toward meaningful objectives is increasingly expected of services whose mission is to focus on active rehabilitation rather than on maintenance or "clinical stability." It therefore is important that objectives be accurate and consistent with each of the characteristics noted below.

> *Beware of the lengthy objectives that use the word 'and' – it often means there are multiple objectives rolled into one. This compromises the measurability of the objective. Each objective should be written to reflect a concrete targeted improvement in ONE specific area.*

- *Behavioral*—observable actions on the part of the service user, specific enough so that the team will know when the objective has been achieved
- *Achievable*—the objective is considered within the reach of the person receiving services within the time frame (although there is no obligation or requirement from accrediting bodies that the objective be met *per se*)
- *Measurable*—that there is some way to quantify the change and answer the question, "Was this objective achieved, yes or no?"
- *Time framed*—with a target date for expected completion
- *Meaningful* and understandable for the person served

There are several methods in the human services field for remembering the technical criteria for well-written objectives. One frequently utilized mnemonic associated with the writing of objectives is the "S-M-A-R-T" acronym. Specifically, this prompts the PCCP plan-writer to ensure that objectives are:

- *S*pecific
- *M*easurable
- *A*ttainable/achievable
- *R*ealistic
- *T*ime framed

When it is unclear whether or not an objective achieves these technical criteria, a simpler strategy for checking on the measurability of this plan element is to read the objective aloud and then ask yourself the question: *As written, will we definitely be able to say YES or NO, that is, was the objective achieved at the end of the time frame, without differences of opinion among the team?* This is perhaps the best litmus test for whether or not an objective is truly focused on concrete and measurable behavioral change. If the objective statement does not meet this standard, chances are it was somehow too subjective or "soft" on the front end and should be revised to reflect the criteria noted above.

In terms of time frames, short-term objectives should be the most active and dynamic part of the PCCP as they reflect the progress that is made toward the specified personal goal. While the longer term goal statement may remain the same over an extended period of time, it is important that objectives be crafted in a way that the individual has a reasonable likelihood of success in achieving them within a shorter time frame, for example, 3 or 6 months, depending on how often the PCCP team is reconvening to review the plan. Increasingly, national standards determine this period of time, that is, funders and accrediting bodies often require that service plans be reviewed at minimum every 90 days. Ideally, the time frame for accomplishment of an objective is 90 days or less—and setting even shorter time frames, that is so-called "low hanging fruit" for "early quick wins," can communicate a message of positive expectation, confidence, and hope for change.

Objectives: A Common Quality Error

> The services, treatments, or supports offered by a practitioner are *not* objectives. They are interventions.

Perhaps the most frequent problem seen in creating a quality written care plan is the confusion between objectives and services or interventions. Objectives should be about meaningful changes in behavior, functioning, or improvement in status—not merely about *service participation!* Attending a group session is NOT the objective—rather the changes the person can make and the benefit derived from participating in such a group is what should be captured and described in the objective statement. For example, it is not uncommon to see a goal such as *I want to have a girlfriend* followed by objectives such as *"Patient will maintain medication compliance, attend social skills group, and meet with his or her therapist weekly,* as if participation in these activities will somehow magically lead to the concrete progress and behavior change that will move the person closer to his or her goal of being in a meaningful relationship. Things such as psychiatric medication, social skills groups, and individual therapy may well be a critical part of the PCCP, but these are interventions, *not* objectives. When crafting the objectives, ask yourself: *As a result of attending the social skills group or using medication effectively, what is the hoped-for change in functioning, behavior, or status?* For example, within a certain time frame, will the person be able to ...

- Identify three places in the local community he or she can go to meet others or identify three positive coping strategies to manage anxiety in social situations (known as a *learning objectives*)
- Participate in one preferred social activity outside the residential setting per week or demonstrate three "conversation starters" in sessions with the clinician, or perhaps actually use those conversation starters to invite someone out on a date! (these are known as *behavioral* objectives as they reflect the application of learning to achieve real behavior change, and as such, they are preferred over "learning" objectives wherever possible)

> **Some wording for objectives**
>
> "Within X days ... The individual will ... "
>   "As a result of services and supports, Mr./Ms. X will ......, as evidenced by ...... "

Finally, objectives that focus on meaningful behavior change rather than defaulting to service participation are necessary both to demonstrate medical necessity and to truly promote recovery. The objective should reflect what needs to change in order for the person to achieve his or her goal, or what action the person will take that is different from before (change in status), such as returning to work by a certain date or perhaps evidencing abstinence from alcohol for a certain time period (in order to meet the goal of "getting my job back"). In contrast, merely "attending" a class, a group, or an individual therapy session does not necessarily indicate a change in the individual's behavior, status, or level of functioning. Sadly, the fact is that many people in this country have faithfully attended services for years, decades even, and never experienced an improvement, in part due to our passive acceptance of service participation as an appropriate short-term outcome. Well-written objectives therefore represent an opportunity to reflect on whether or not the plan is working to help the person take legitimate steps forward in their recovery. In this way, the review of objectives can become a useful part of routine services as practitioner and service user together reflect on the progress made (or not) toward the short-term objectives, *"Ok, since our last meeting, where did you hope you'd be in terms of getting back to work? Have you achieved that short-term objective? If not, why not? Are there additional services that would be helpful, or personal action steps you had a hard time following through on? What would be helpful in getting back on track?"*

In summary, while the crafting of objectives involves perhaps the most stringent of technical criteria from a documentation perspective, they can also serve to maximize the person-centered dimensions of the care plan as they communicate positive expectations for change while mapping out concrete next steps on the path to recovery and wellness.

Interventions

Finally, we consider the final element of the person-centered care plan, the interventions section, also referred to as the *methods* or *services* section. While professional services are certainly an essential part of the plan, a high-quality, comprehensive PCCP also includes within the interventions section any action steps or tasks that will be owned, and acted on by, unpaid natural supporters or the person himself or herself. This is consistent with the emphasis that PCCP places on maximizing both personal responsibility and self-agency as well as the individual's connections to natural support relationships. Traditional treatment plans often limit this section of the planning document to reflect only those treatments that clinical, rehabilitation, medical, and other professionals are paid to deliver. This method of completing the interventions section can lead to PCCPs that read as a laundry list of all of the "treatments" that are going to be done to (or for) the person while missing out on a key opportunity to capitalize on the resources and talents of the person himself or herself as well as other members of his or her support network.

As with the approach to actively incorporating strengths in the PCCP document, when the preplanning process has uncovered persons within the support network who are willing, and able, to lend their time, energy, and enthusiasm to the person's PCCP vision, these contributions should be documented as action steps alongside those services offered by professional practitioners. Similarly, documenting an action step (which may be as ambitious or as modest as needed) for the person to take primary responsibility is an important opportunity to build a sense of self-agency and move past the legacy of passivity and low expectations that has unfortunately become common among persons with disabilities involved in professional service systems.

Types of Interventions

Within the PCCP process, the team should explore a diverse array of professional services, alternative strategies, and natural supports to assist the person in realizing his or her PCCP vision. Some examples include:

- Professionally delivered clinical interventions such as medications or psychotherapy, including evidence-based practices when applicable.
- Self-help and peer support.
- Exercise and nutrition guidance.
- Rehabilitation and skill-building to enable the person to live in the least restrictive environment.
- Daily maintenance activities and plans for managing symptoms and behaviors before they get worse (e.g., Wellness Recovery Action Plans).
- Spiritual practices and affiliations.
- Homeopathic and naturopathic remedies.
- Cultural healing practices/involvement of indigenous healers.
- Increased involvement in community activities or connections with natural supporters.
- Rehabilitation opportunities such as supported housing, supported education, supported employment, and supported community living.
- Practical assistance in community contexts to address basic human needs for housing, food, work, and connection with the community.

It is essential that interventions reflect the choices and preferences of the individual. While it may seem like common sense to just ask the person what he or she prefers, the "interventions" listed on most treatment plans still typically reflect only what is commonly available within the system or agency and not what the person's preference for support may be. To make sure the plan is truly person-directed, practitioners should ask questions about how the person wants to pursue his or her hopes, dreams, interests, and aspirations in addition to what is perhaps the most important question of all: "How can I best be of help to you?"

Addressing Regulatory and Fiscal Pressures in Writing Interventions

When it comes to documenting services and supports that will be billed to a medical insurer—very commonly Medicaid—it is important that the intervention be recorded in a way that the essential information necessary to meet the regulatory requirements is included. In order to clearly demonstrate the medical necessity of a service or support activity, the intervention should include and specify each of the five critical elements:

- practitioner and clinical/professional discipline;
- staff member's name (wherever possible, recognizing that in some team-based service models, there may be multiple individuals called on to deliver a certain support);

- modality of the intervention or service, for example, group therapy, case management, rehab services, nutritional counseling;
- frequency (how often?, for example, 2 times per month); intensity (how long?, for example, for 30 min); duration (over what period of time? for example, for 3 months);
- purpose, intent, and anticipated impact.

The medical necessity of the proposed activity will be clear so long as the purpose of the intervention in helping the individual attain the objective is specified. The clearer the link between the activity and the desired change in the objective, the clearer the case for medical necessity. A helpful strategy for checking to ensure you have maintained the logical link between the objective and the intervention is to read the plan from the "bottom-up"—meaning, read the interventions and then go back and read the objective statement. If the logical link is not apparent, this may have just been an oversight in the documentation and the practitioner can now revise the plan. However, if the purpose of the interventions is frequently unclear and/or seemingly unrelated to the attainment of objectives on the PCCP, this can be an indication that service users are simply assigned to a daily or weekly series of interventions/groups because this is "what we offer here." This would be an example of a system-centered program design where individuals fit into the available service menu and goals are developed after verifying facts; in essence, the plan jumps right to interventions without adequate attention to person-centered goals and objective setting. In a high-quality PCCP process, the team works together to design the interventions around the person and not the other way around!

A Note on Evidenced-Based Practices in the Person-Centered Plan

In thinking about interventions, it is essential to recognize the growing emphasis on providing services that have an evidence base that demonstrates their effectiveness. These types of "evidence-based" services should be considered in the development of the plan and clearly explained to the focus person. It is the responsibility of administrators and service practitioners to be familiar with these practices and to ensure that they are available as options within a range of interventions from which the focus person can choose. Detailed information and resources regarding evidence-based practices (also referred to as *EBPs*) can be accessed at www.mentalhealth.samhsa.gov/cmhs/communitysupport/toolkits/.

While EBPs have been shown to work for certain people under certain research and life conditions, for a given length of time, they are not the *only* interventions that can positively impact a person's recovery. There are many "values-based" and "experience-based" approaches (e.g., culturally specific interventions, peer-based programming, faith-based approaches) that have not yet been studied as extensively in academic settings but have been found by many people to be highly effective. These are generally termed *emerging* or *promising* practices, and often they are practices associated with recovery-oriented systems change. Additional information on this topic is provided in both the Federal Mental Health Action Agenda [5] and the What Helps ... What Hinders report [6]. The exploration and use of both evidence-based practices and emerging or promising practices is an important part of PCCP.

In summary, clearly documenting the intended purpose of the service provided is an opportunity to improve the PCCP from a "compliance" perspective. However, it is an equally important opportunity to "connect the dots" and to demonstrate to the individual that the provision of services has stayed true to the goals and objectives in which he or she has expressed interest. For example, will I be meeting with a psychiatrist for the purpose of discussing the side effects of medications on sexual life, which may interfere with my goal of getting a girlfriend? Or will I be meeting with the psychiatrist so that he or she can check off the boxes on the follow-up forms that are required for him or her to secure reimbursement for my care? Similar questions can be asked about other domains of practice. Will I be meeting with the money manager for the purpose of learning skills so that I can manage my money as I move out of the group home or because the staff do not approve of how I spend my money? Will I be meeting with a therapist for the purpose of developing communication skills that will help me to be a better parent or because the staff think that I "have issues"? When the individualized purpose of the intervention is described in this way, the person is far more likely to see the intended benefit as it relates to his or her personal PCCP vision.

Putting the Pieces Together: A Sample PCCP Excerpt for Juliet

Introducing Juliet

Juliet is a 22-year-old female who dreams of finishing school and becoming a preschool teacher someday. She has been receiving mental health services since she was 16 in order to help her manage major depression and periods of hallucinations. The confusion and voices tend to become much worse when she is depressed or "stressed out." She moved from Texas to Massachusetts 1 year ago hoping for a fresh start. Against her mother's advice, she enrolled in local Adult Ed classes and soon felt overwhelmed with the demands. She experienced severe anxiety, her voices became much worse, and she was eventually hospitalized. Juliet is transferred to your caseload six months after this hospitalization, and she seems to enjoy talking with you. After several meetings with her, you find that she would like to begin to take classes again. She had a good relationship with her primary academic advisor who was aware of, and supportive around, her mental health issues. However, Juliet's mom is against her returning to school at this time and she has urged her not to rush things, and to take more time to "get things straight." Juliet does acknowledge that she is still experiencing voices, but she is learning how to cope with them and feels much more relaxed in recent months. Previous severe sleep disturbance is significantly improved (Juliet achieved an earlier objective on her recovery plan targeting this issue), and she feels she is ready to take the next step toward her goal of finishing school and being a teacher.

Figure 6.3 is an excerpt of a sample person-centered care plan based on Juliet's story. Note how the goal begins with, and is driven by, Juliet's stated goal to resume her education so she can become a school teacher. However, it also simultaneously acknowledges some of the significant mental health barriers that are interfering with this goal and documents multiple services and supports she can draw on to overcome them. We leave you with this example to demonstrate how the pieces of a PCCP come together, thereby giving you hope that it is, in fact, possible to create a plan that both honors the person AND satisfies the chart!

> **Goal:**
> *I want to get my degree in education and be a teacher someday.*

<table>
<tr>
<td>

Strengths & Resources

Support of her instructors around her mental health issues; close relationship with her mother; Juliet understands her illness and what tends to trigger an increase in symptoms; very motivated to move forward on her goal of working as a school teacher; friendly and outgoing personality, connects well with others, including staff at the mental health center.

</td>
<td>

Barriers/Needs That Interfere

Increase in voices around the stress of attending classes; sleep disturbance due to stress & major depression; lack of support from her mother around attending school; difficulty concentrating; previously unable to meet attendance requirements at GED class due to high anxiety; difficulty remembering, tracking, and completing assignments; anxiety related to taking bus to GED classes

</td>
</tr>
</table>

> **Short-term Objective:**
> *Over the next 90 days, Juliet will self-report missing no more than 4 of her GED classes at the Adult Ed Department due to anxiety or oversleeping.*

> **Interventions & Action Steps:**
>
> • Alan Elihu, M.D., will provide medication management 1x monthly for 3 months for the purpose of minimizing distressing symptoms which interfere with school performance, anxiety, sleep disturbance, cognitive issues, etc.
>
> • Deborah Brick, L.C.S.W., will provide 1:1 cognitive behavioral therapy 1x weekly for 3 months to assist with stress management and teach positive coping skills.
>
> • Joan Ainsely, R.N., will provide education in sleep hygiene skills 1x weekly for 3 months in order to expand self-management tools/strategies to maintain healthy sleep habits/patterns.
>
> • Jesse Iwanski, Peer Specialist, will meet with Juliet 3xs over next 4 weeks to assist her in creating a Wellness Recovery Action Plan, in order to help her manage stress and maintain wellness.
>
> • Althea Jackson, Supported Education Specialist, will meet with Juliet and representative of Adult Ed Special Services Department a minimum of one time monthly over the next 3 months for the purpose of coordinating services and helping Juliet to arrange necessary classroom accommodations.
>
> • Juliet's mom has agreed to ride the bus with Juliet during her first month of GED class to help ease this source of anxiety and ensure a smooth transition.
>
> • Juliet will practice a minimum of 3 of her WRAP wellness activities on a daily basis to manage anxiety as she transitions back to class.

Figure 6.3   Sample PCCP for Juliet

Exercises

Exercise 1. Personal PCCP Planning

Think about the material covered in this Module—the conceptual definition of each distinct plan component as well as the relationship *between* the components. Respond to each of the questions below on a separate piece of paper as a way to practice and apply your learning.

- Identify one of your important personal goals.
- What are some of the strengths, skills, and resources you possess to move you toward this goal?
- What are some of the barriers, what gets in the way?
- Write a time framed, measurable objective for your goal.
- Who can help you in achieving this goal?
- What was it like to go through this process for one of your own goals?
- What would it be like for someone to tell you to put this goal "on hold" because they were concerned you are "not ready?"
- How might this inform or change how you carry out PCCP with a person receiving services?

Exercise 2. Writing Measurable Objectives

Each of the following objectives has one or more elements missing. Take the following objectives and

1. Identify what's missing or unclear—is there an identified time frame? Is the objective behavioral? Is it something that can be measured?
2. Rewrite them so that they contain all the required technical elements: they should
   - Build on strengths and resources
   - Be time framed
   - Be meaningful and understandable for the person served
   - And, be
     - Behavioral
     - Achievable
     - Measurable
3. Refer to the sample answers at the end of the Module for ideas on rewriting objectives.

Note: Some examples may need to have the content changed, others will just need to have more specifics added. There is no one right way to complete this exercise—be creative!

1. Client will decrease social isolation.
2. Shonda will increase her level of physical exercise as a way to help with her depression.
3. Client will reduce assaultive behavior.
4. Client will decrease the frequency and intensity of substance use.
5. Client will comply with money management plan for the next 3 months.
6. Ron will verbally identify the coping strategies.
7. Jeanie's diabetes will be better controlled within 90 days.
8. Joe will attend Med-Ed group regularly over the next 30 days.
9. Ann will use relaxation techniques to improve sleep within 90 days.
10. Luis will carry out ADLs independently in 6 months.

Exercise 3. Putting the Pieces Together in a Person-Centered Plan: Mr. Blake

We present a set of assessment data and person-centered narrative summary for Mr. Blake. After reading the material, attempt to write a PCCP excerpt that will get Mr. Blake closer to one of his valued recovery goals. Write ONE goal, a set of strengths and barriers, a short-term objective (according to the S-M-A-R-T criteria), and a diverse set of interventions/actions steps (including those owned by Mr. Blake and/or his natural supporters). After you have completed this task, review the sample person-centered plan provided for Mr. Blake at the conclusion of this module, and consider the following questions:

- How did your plan for Mr. Blake compare? Did you have similar ideas for goals and objectives or did you take the plan in a different direction? [Remember—there is no ONE "right" way to write a person-centered plan. Samples are provided only for the sake of illustration and to promote the discussion of ideas.]
- Were goal statements in Mr. Blake's own words?
- How did you actively incorporate his strengths into the goals, objectives, or interventions?
- Did your short-term objective hold up to the S-M-A-R-T criteria? Would it feel meaningful for Mr. Blake and move him closer to his long-term goal and his desire for independence?
- Did you include all the necessary components in documenting mental health services, that is, WHO is doing it (practitioner name or role), WHAT are they doing (service type or modality), WHEN are they doing it (schedule), and WHY—for what reason (purpose/intent/impact)?
- Did you include an action step for Mr. Blake and/or his natural supporters or was the interventions section limited to those services provided by professional practitioners?

Mr. Blake's Assessment

Identifying Information, Presenting Concerns, and Living Situation

Mr. Blake is a 33-year-old African American male who has been living in a shared-apartment program with residential and clinical supports for 12 months following years of intermittent homelessness and repeated psychiatric hospitalizations. Now he is enjoying his single longest period of being successfully housed in the community as an adult, and though he is proud of this achievement, he wants to move to an apartment of his own and is ready to start making steps toward that goal. He reports being much more comfortable in a private space, and he has become increasingly upset about the pace of the transition. Currently, Mr. Blake has frequent visits from various staff who monitor his status, manage his money, and deliver his medications twice daily. But, he wants to move to his own scattered-site apartment (without a roommate or onsite case management) where he would have greater privacy and independence. As he has become more dissatisfied with his progress, he started missing visits from his Medication Monitor as well as the Benefits Specialist who helps manage his money. Staff met with Mr. Blake to discuss their concerns, but Mr. Blake reports that things were "fine." He is just tired of other people controlling "my money, my meds, and my life." He agrees that there were certain things he needs to work on in order to succeed in an apartment of his own, and he says he wants to develop a recovery plan that will help move him closer to that goal.

Strengths

Mr. Blake reports that his biggest strengths are having a strong work ethic and "never giving up on myself." He has a natural talent for "fixing things," and reports that he is most calm when he is busy with his hands. Despite a long history of disconnection from the mental health system, Mr. Blake is now connected to both residential and clinical services and he is willing to work with staff once he is convinced that they are helping him gain some independence in his life.

Mental Health Concerns and Service History

Written records and the report of family members (mother and cousin) suggest that Mr. Blake was exhibiting signs of severe depression, social isolation, and strange behaviors in his late teens and early twenties. However, Mr. Blake did not have his first full-blown psychotic break and hospitalization until the age of 24 after the sudden death of his infant son from an undiagnosed heart defect. The child—the product of a brief relationship in his early twenties—regularly visited Mr. Blake at the apartment he shared with his mother until the child died suddenly while in his care at the age of 10 months. Mr. Blake was unable to wake the child from a nap, and his attempts to resuscitate the baby were unsuccessful. Autopsy indicated his son passed from an undiagnosed heart defect, but Mr. Blake became convinced that someone in the building had killed the child through poisoning and that he had failed to protect the child. He was hospitalized after he threatened and punched a neighbor whom he had accused of being involved in the death. Mr. Blake's mother and cousin report that he never fully recovered from this loss, and that the event started off nearly a decade of psychiatric instability, repeated hospitalizations, and periods of homelessness.

Mr. Blake has had difficulty living independently in the community as cognitive disorganization has led him to neglect basic household or personal care tasks and symptoms of paranoia have led to frequent conflicts with others. He often believes that neighbors in the community are intent on harming him, and when this occurs, he becomes isolative—refusing to leave his apartment or open his door to anyone. He has also previously been evicted from two apartment complexes for making repeated calls to the police/emergency services to report he "fears for his life" and to make unsubstantiated accusations regarding various neighbors—behaviors that are typically followed by hospitalizations or periods of homelessness. Currently, Mr. Blake is being treated for symptoms associated with a diagnosis of schizophrenia. He experiences paranoia, depressive mood disturbance, and cognitive issues such as difficulty with organizing and concentrating on tasks.

Family and Social Support History

Mr. Blake was an only child raised by a single-parent mother who worked two jobs to support the family. He never had a relationship with his father who, he learned in his teenage years, was incarcerated repeatedly for drug-related offenses. Mr. Blake spent a great deal of time with his aunt and a cousin, Ronnie, who lived in their apartment building while he was growing up. He was an average student until his Junior year of high school when he began to experience what he describes as "anxiety" because he "never fit in." He began avoiding relationships and activities, and by the fall of his Senior year, Mr. Blake stopped attending all classes, and he was unable to graduate from high school. He began attending outpatient services at the local mental health clinic where he was briefly treated for depression before he stopped participating in further treatment despite the pleas of his mother. Mr. Blake stopped taking care of himself, and increasingly spent most of the day sleeping in his room at home, going out only occasionally to wander the streets or to pick up odd jobs in the neighborhood.

Despite his mental health difficulties and hospitalizations, Mr. Blake has stayed in touch with his cousin who comes over regularly to watch basketball games. He also describes his mother as supportive, although he has recently been arguing with her because she does not want him to move to an apartment of his own because she is afraid of what is going to happen. Mr. Blake's relationship with his mother has been strained since the death of his son nearly a decade ago (see Mental Health Section). Mr. Blake had been living with his mother at the time of this event, and she did not agree with Mr. Blake's theory that a neighbor poisoned the baby, and Mr. Blake believed she supported a cover-up of the "murder" of his son. Furthermore, she would not allow Mr. Blake to return to her home after his hospitalization unless he agreed to get intensive mental health treatment that he did not pursue for several years. At several points during this time, he showed up at her home and police needed to be called after he became agitated and threatened her. They have recently reconnected through mail and telephone contact while Mr. Blake has been living in the shared-apartment program. Mr. Blake would like to rebuild his relationship with his mother and his mother too shares this desire.

Mr. Blake also has a positive relationship with the owner of a local thrift-goods store. The owner has looked out for Mr. Blake for several years, giving him blankets and necessities when he was living on the streets and paying him to do odd jobs around the store as needed. Mr. Blake acknowledges that he has difficulty going out of the house or meeting new people because of his "nerves" and he wishes he were able to be comfortable around others and do some of the activities he used to enjoy as a teen, playing basketball, going to movies with friends, listening to music, and so on.

Medication Information

After years of inconsistent use of medications, recently, Mr. Blake has responded well to a combination of fluoxetine and risperidone to treat symptoms of depression and psychosis. Though he has been taking these medications consistently for the past 10 months, he does not talk openly about his meds or his illness other than to say that he "gets nervous when people mess with" him and that the meds keep him "calm" when he is not doing good. He says he will continue to take the medications, but is very frustrated with "waiting around for the nurse to come twice a day." He wants to be more independent in taking his medications. He also reports feeling like a "zombie" at times and he wants his meds adjusted so that he is not so fatigued because he would like to get back to doing odd jobs around the neighborhood and looking for part-time work.

Risk/Safety

Mr. Blake does not report any suicidal or homicidal ideation and is not currently considered to be a risk to himself or others. Though he continues to believe that people sometimes "mess with" *him, he is willing to learn alternative coping strategies to manage stress and/or interpersonal problems when he is feeling unsafe.*

Health Summary

Mr. Blake does not have any significant medical issues requiring attention.

Legal Status and Legal History

Mr. Blake has no current legal problems.

Community Living Skills and Housing Issues

Mr. Blake had limited experience living on his own or maintaining a household until his recent experience in the shared-apartment program. Residential Counselors report that he gets very disorganized and does not follow a routine to take care of his responsibilities—including paying his bills and household chores. He tends to spend a lot of time in his bedroom, watching TV and fixing small electronics that he finds in neighborhood dumpsters and repairs them to make money. When he has lived in apartments in the past, he has become suspicious of neighbors and does not have the inclination to participate in any community activities as a result of these feelings.

Employment and Education

Mr. Blake was unable to finish high school due to his mental health issues, but during a period of relative mental health stability 3 years ago, he was able to complete his GED with the help of a tutor at a local psychosocial rehabilitation program. Mr. Blake describes himself as a hard worker, and his mother reports that he could "fix anything as a kid" and has a natural aptitude for hands-on work. Mr. Blake confirms that he is most "at peace" when he is working on fixing things.

Finances and Benefits

Mr. Blake is currently receiving supplemental security income (SSI) benefits. His money is managed by staff at his shared-apartment residential program, and he is given a minimal weekly allowance. He tends to spend his funds the first few days he has them, and then resorts to panhandling or requesting loans from his neighbors in order to get by until his next allocation. He would like greater control of his money but admits he has little experience with managing his finances or paying the types of bills that will be associated with a move to an apartment of his own.

Mr. Blake: Person-Centered Narrative Summary

Mr. Blake values his independence and speaks up for what is important to him. Over the past decade, he has demonstrated remarkable resilience surviving highly distressing psychiatric symptoms, the traumatic loss of a child, and extended periods of homelessness. Through all these experiences, he maintained a positive connection to a cousin as well as a local thrift-shop owner. Mr. Blake also describes his mother as being an important source of support, though their relationship has been strained at times as he has struggled with his mental health issues and impairments associated with a diagnosis of paranoid schizophrenia.

In the past 12 months, Mr. Blake has successfully been living in a shared-apartment program with clinical and residential services. This represents his single longest period of time living in the community as an adult, and it is a significant change from what has been a long history of distrust and disconnection from formal mental health services. Though he is proud of this achievement, he wants to move to a "scattered-site" apartment of his own where he will have more privacy and control over his life, finances, and medications.

The team would like to support this decision but staff is concerned regarding Mr. Blake's ability to manage his medications, his budget/finances, and his relationships with new neighbors. He has continued to experience persistent symptoms of both paranoia and cognitive confusion while living in the shared-apartment program over the past year, and, in their opinion, Mr. Blake, has not yet developed the skills and coping strategies he will need in order to manage these symptoms and succeed in a lower level of care. He tends to minimize the impairments he experiences, and he sees the world as a dangerous place—a perception that is further complicated by the unresolved issues of grief and loss over the death of his son, for example, "There is nothing wrong with me. People just have it in for me." At the same time, he has made significant progress in the past year in beginning to discuss his "nerves" and how he feels uncomfortable around other people or sometimes gets confused and neglects things around the house. He has been taking medications consistently and has generally been making use of services offered to him. He vacillates between the contemplation and action stage of change but is willing to participate in programming that will move him closer to his goal of living and working in the community as independently as possible. Mr. Blake has many strengths to draw upon, including a strong work ethic, enduring natural support relationships, an improved relationship with his treatment team, an ability to learn and complete tasks (e.g., persisting to achieve his GED), and a desire to be more independent and to reconnect with preferred community activities, as he works toward these goals.

Learning Assessment

Module 6: Documentation of PCCP: Writing the Plan to Honor the person AND Satisfy the Chart		
Statement	True	False
1. A goal is a simple statement of what a person wants to achieve.		
2. It is important for goals to be realistic so that people are not set up for disappointment.		
3. S-M-A-R-T objectives are short-term medication and recovery treatment steps.		
4. Interventions are done to a person for their safety.		
5. Actions taken by the service user and his/her natural supporters should be documented in the recovery plan alongside those services provided by professional staff.		
See the Answer Key at the end of chapter for the correct answers. **Number Correct**		
0 to 2: Don't be discouraged. Learning is an ongoing process! You can review the Module for greater knowledge. 3 to 4: You have a solid foundation. Use this Module to enhance your skills. 5: You are ahead of the game! Use this Module to teach others and strive for excellence!		

References

1. Department of Health and Human Services. (2003) *Achieving the Promise. Transforming Mental Health Care in America*. Substance Abuse and Mental Health Services Administration, Rockville, MD.
2. Adams N, Grieder D. (2005). *Treatment Planning for Person-Centered Care: The Road to Mental Health and Addiction Recovery*. Elsevier Academic Press, San Diego, CA.
3. Tondora J, O'Connell M, Dinzeo T *et al.* (2010) A clinical trial of peer-based culturally responsive person-centered care for psychosis for African Americans and Latinos. *Clinical Trials* 7, 368–379.
4. Sa'adi. (2007) *Gulistan (The Rose Garden)*. Translated by Edwin Arthur. Cosimo: New York, NY.
5. Department of Health and Human Services. (2005) *Transforming Mental Health Care in America: An Action Plan*. Substance Abuse and Mental Health Services Administration, Rockville, MD.
6. Onken SJ, Dumont JM, Ridgway P *et al.* (2002) *Mental Health Recovery: What Helps and What Hinders? A National Research Project for the Development of Recovery Facilitating System Performance Indicators. Phase One Research Report*. National Association of State Mental Health Program Directors National Technical Assistance Center, Alexandria, VA.

Writing Measurable Objectives

1. Client will decrease social isolation.
   - *Larissa will increase her social network over the next 3 months as evidenced by attending a minimum of 1 event per week with a friend or family member.*
2. Shonda will increase her level of physical exercise as a way to help with her depression.
   - *For the next 90 days, Shonda will increase her level of physical exercise as evidenced by the self-report of walking 3 times a week for 15 min each time.*
3. Client will reduce assaultive behavior.
   - *Within 90 days, Amy will verbally identify 3 triggers that have led to physical altercations with her children* (an example of a more modest learning-oriented objective). Or,
   - *Within 90 days, Amy will have a minimum of one successful visit with her children as evidenced by the report of her Child Protective Services worker* (an example of a more ambitious behavior-change objective).
4. Client will decrease the frequency and intensity of substance use.
   - *Joe will identify a minimum of two adverse effects that substance use has on his/her recovery within 30 days* (e.g., if Joe is in early precontemplative stage of change). Or,
   - *Joe will be substance-free for 6 months as evidenced by self-report* (if Joe is more action-oriented)
5. Client will comply with money management plan for the next 3 months.
   - *Gary will open a savings account within 2 weeks.* Or,
   - *Gary will successfully manage his money over the next months as evidenced by zero reports of panhandling from staff or other residents.* Or,
   - *Within 6 months, Gary will have saved enough money to go on a bus trip with his daughter.*
6. Ron will verbally identify coping strategies.
   - *Ron will verbally identify a minimum of three positive coping strategies to clinician within the next 2 weeks* (an example of a more modest learning-oriented objective). Or,
   - *Ron will apply positive coping strategies to take the bus independently a minimum of three times over the next month* (an example of a more ambitious behavior-change objective).
7. Jeanie's diabetes will be better controlled within 90 days.
   - *Within 90 days Jeanie's diabetes will be better controlled as evidenced by her daily readings on her glucometer at 200 or less.*
8. Joe will attend Med-Ed group regularly over the next 30 days.
   - *Joe will verbally note the therapeutic impact of each of his medications to the Group leader within 30 days.* Or,
   - *Joe will demonstrate ability to accurately self-administer his morning medications as evidenced by his nurse observations within 90 days.*
9. Ann will use relaxation techniques to improve sleep within 90 days.
   - *Within 90 days, Ann will sleep a minimum of 6 h per night at least 6 days per week as evidenced by her sleep log.*

10. Luis will carry out ADLs independently within 6 months.
    ◦ *Within 6 months, Luis will correctly balance his checkbook for 3 consecutive months as evidenced by the report of Benefits Specialist.*

Mr. Blake's Sample Recovery Plan for Comparison

Three Possible Recovery Plan Excerpts

Note: Three separate recovery goal areas are identified for illustrating diversity in the type of plan goals and content that might be included for Mr. Blake. There are *many* possible ways that a quality recovery plan might come together. For example, depending on actual circumstances and preferences, Mr. Blake's plan may have only included one of the three noted goal areas presented below. Another alternative might be to organize the plan around the overarching long-term goal of independent apartment living with certain components integrated underneath this goal as shorter term objectives. Any of these structures can be appropriate provided they are mutually negotiated in partnership with the person-in recovery—there is no single "right" way to develop a person-centered plan!

Goal #1

"I want control of my money back."

Strengths

Recognizes the need for skill development; basic math skills are intact; family is willing to assist.

Barriers/Assessed Needs

Mr. Blake has limited experience budgeting and paying his own bills. Cognitive and depressive symptoms have also led Mr. Blake to neglect bills in the past, and the failure to pay his rent has resulted in eviction proceedings. Mr. Blake has difficulty planning ahead and overspending has also led to panhandling and multiple requests for loans from the residential program. Budgeting skill level has led to *weekly* allocations of funds that Mr. Blake objects to.

Objectives

1. Mr. Blake will successfully budget a *monthly* personal allowance over the next 6 months as evidenced by the report of Residential Counselor that Mr. Blake has been able to pay bills and meet expenses without loan requests.

Interventions and Action Steps

1. Mary Tomason, Benefits Coordinator, to provide weekly, 60-minute skill-building group for the next 6 months in order to build personal budgeting skills and to provide support as Mr. Blake assumes greater control of his money.
2. Anthony Sells, M.D., to provide medication evaluation and monitoring two times per month for 30 min for the next 3 months for purposes of decreasing symptoms and maximizing cognitive functioning, including his ability to manage his own funds and attend to bills.
3. *Mr. Blake will gather all bills and records of expenses within one week in order to inform the modified budget he will be working on with Benefits Coordinator. (Self-directed action)*
4. *Mr. Jansen, thrift-shop owner, has agreed to purchase a calculator for Mr. Blake within one week for use in his budgeting efforts. (Natural support action)*

Goal #2

"I want to manage my meds on my own. I am tired of waiting around for the nurse all day."

Strengths

Strong family support; increasing recognition that the meds help with "nerves" and feeling uncomfortable around other people; consistent use of medications in the past 10 months when delivered by staff nurse and prompted; desire to learn and be more independent with med self-administration.

Barriers/Assessed Needs

Cognitive symptoms lead to forgetfulness in taking meds; can become disorganized and have difficulty accurately identifying pills and correct dosages; concerns regarding the side effect of fatigue may contribute to inconsistent use of medications; baseline med administration skills has led to two daily visits from the visiting nurse, which Mr. Blake would like to reduce.

Objective

Within 3 months, Mr. Blake will demonstrate the ability to accurately self-administer his afternoon dose of psychiatric medications on five consecutive visits as evidenced by nursing services report.*

Interventions and Action Steps

1. Rashida Waters, Medication Coordinator, to provide twice monthly medication education for 30 min for the next 3 months in order to assist Mr. Blake in the effective use of

medications to decrease symptoms and to address evaluate/address any of his concerns regarding side effects (e.g., fatigue).

2. Sam Narrato, Peer Coordinator, to provide twice weekly, 45-min Meds & Me group for 3 months in order to assist Mr. Blake in becoming more informed about his meds and more comfortable talking with his doctor/nurse about any concerns/questions he may have.

3. Connie Clayton, Clinic Therapist, to provide individual therapy 45 min weekly for the next 3 months in order to assist Mr. Blake and the visiting nurse with identifying barriers and developing compensatory strategies for med self-administration.

4. *Mr. Blake will purchase a pill box within one week so he can use this to better organize his daily meds and dosages with the visiting nurse. (Self-directed action)*

5. *Susan Jackson, Local Rights and Advocacy Coordinator, will offer a monthly 60-min workshop, Finding Your Voice: Completing and Using Your Psychiatric Advance Directive, until Mr. Blake has finalized a PAD that allows him to indicate his preferences and plan ahead for any potential psychiatric crisis as he assumes greater control of his medications. (Community support action)*

* Note: Achievement of this objective will prompt discontinuation of PM nursing visit at which point Mr. Blake's cousin, Ronnie, has agreed to text him every afternoon from work to remind him to take his meds.

Goal #3

"I don't want to be alone anymore. I want to have friends and family in my life."

Strengths

Long history of a successful and close relationship with his cousin and positive connection to a local thrift-shop owner; after years of social isolation, Mr. Blake is expressing interest in reconnecting with his mother, making friends in his apartment building, and trying new activities

Barriers/Assessed Needs

Mr. Blake feels very uncomfortable around others and often believes people are out to harm him in some way; needs coping skills; has made calls to police in the past when feeling unsafe; behaves in a manner that others perceive as "odd" and defensive; conflicts with his mother over their differing views of his mental illness and the death of his son; social isolation and fears of others prevent Mr. Blake from leaving the house for regular social activities

Objectives

1. Mr. Blake will participate in a minimum of two social activities per week outside his home each week for the next 3 months as evidenced by the report of the Residential Counselor.

Interventions

1. Jane Arsenal, Clinician, will provide Trauma-Informed Individual Therapy, 2x per month for 45 minutes for next 3 mos for the purpose of supporting Mr. Blake in processing the loss and trauma around the death of son and educating him regarding the event's impact on his relationships with others.
2. Jerry Angelica, Rehab Coordinator, to provide twice weekly, 60-minute social skills group for the next 3 months in order to assist Mr. Blake in becoming more comfortable in social situations.
3. Ed Manning, Community Integration Coordinator, will provide twice monthly, 90-min Community Connections group for the next 3 months in order to help Mr. Blake identify and access social and recreational outings that fit with his preferred interests and that allow him opportunities to practice social skills in vivo.
4. Sam Narrato, Peer Coordinator, will meet with Mr. Blake once weekly for 60 min for the next 2 months to assist him in completing a Wellness Recovery Action Plan in order to identify simple, safe, effective strategies for managing distressing symptoms that lead to social isolation.
5. Sally Rodriquez, Clinical Coordinator, to provide twice monthly 60-min family session for 6 months to Mr. Blake and his mother, in order to assist them in rebuilding their relationship and in exploring ways Mr. Blake and his mother can spend time together.
6. *Mr. Blake will call his mother within one week to invite her to meet with Sally Rodriguez, Clinical Coordinator. (Self-directed action)*
7. *Ronnie P., Mr. Blake's cousin, has agreed to accompany him to the monthly potluck dinners in his housing complex so that he can have an opportunity to meet new people and practice coping and social skills. (Natural support action)*

Answers to the Learning Assessment:

1. T
2. F
3. F
4. F
5. T

Module 7: So you have a person-centered care plan, now what? Plan implementation and quality monitoring

Goal

This module focuses on the processes of documentation follow-up, and continuous quality improvement (CQI) after the plan itself is completed. It outlines the key elements necessary to include in a progress note, the practice of charting to the plan, and using the plan as an everyday part of the direct care work. It also focuses on promoting accountability and ongoing consumer satisfaction with person-centered care planning (PCCP) processes and service outcomes. It is intended to help practitioners, administrators, and supervisors to work collaboratively and effectively with individuals to evaluate both the process and the impact of PCCPs.

Learning Objectives

After completing this module, you will be able to:

- identify the key elements and the importance of a progress note in person-centered approaches;
- learn about different structures of writing a progress note;
- understand the value of utilizing the person-centered plan to guide everyday practice;
- understand the definition and benefits of concurrent documentation;
- identify strategies to solicit active service user involvement in ongoing CQI initiatives;
- identify workforce development needs and recovery-specific competencies.

Learning Assessment

A learning assessment is included at the end of the module. If you are already familiar with this subject, you may want to go to the end of this module and take the assessment to see

Partnering for Recovery in Mental Health: A Practical Guide to Person-Centered Planning, First Edition.
Janis Tondora, Rebecca Miller, Mike Slade and Larry Davidson.
© 2014 John Wiley & Sons, Ltd. Published 2014 by John Wiley & Sons, Ltd.

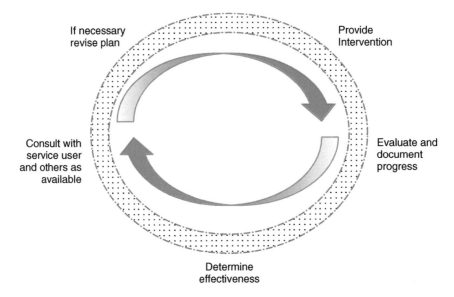

If necessary revise plan

Provide Intervention

Consult with service user and others as available

Evaluate and document progress

Determine effectiveness

Figure 7.1   Cyclical Path for Developing, Implementing, and Revising Care Plan

how much you already know. Then you can focus your learning efforts on what is new for you.

Charting to the Plan

So you and the person you are working with have collaborated with your team to develop a person-centered care plan (PCCP). The document is complete and signed, with all parties agreeing on the respective roles they have to play in promoting the person's recovery. What now? Often times, this is when the plan is filed in a chart and forgotten until 90 days or 6 months have passed, after which it is unearthed and revisited only to be rewritten and filed all over again. The document itself is "dead," with no life, value, or function in your everyday work of assisting people in moving toward their goals, hopes, and dreams (Figure 7.1).

A person-centered process should ideally result, instead, in a plan that can function as a roadmap, a tool that is referred to often as a guide for anticipating what the next steps moving forward entail. Having the plan function as a live and active reference point can sometimes require a dramatic change in process and practice, as this may not be the way many practitioners are accustomed to working. And if it requires a change for practitioners, then it will also require a change for those receiving services as well. Making this shift requires education for all involved, and a thoughtful process of reviewing and revising practices as we move toward the person-centered ideal of using the plan as a roadmap for everyday life.

As with any trip, though, it is important to check in on our progress: Are we on the right road? Do we need to change direction? Are there other people we might need to invite along to help us navigate the next leg of the journey? Part of this assessment is included in the documentation recorded at each meeting when interventions are being provided and the work and progress being made by the person receiving services is reviewed.

As a mental health practitioner you are no doubt familiar with progress or encounter notes, the documentation of each contact or service provided for a person receiving services. What follows here is a brief note on the purpose of progress notes, which may be more of a review but might also provide a new rationale for the note-taking process. Documentation in the clinical record is an integral part of providing mental health services. Though it may seem obvious *why* it is important, we briefly review here several of the reasons that charting is an essential, if perhaps underappreciated, component of providing person-centered care.

Progress notes are an integral part of the PCCP process. A strongly and clearly written plan directly informs the tasks to be achieved as well as the progress notes to be written. In this way, the plan is an integral part of services and their documentation. To write a note, it is necessary to refer back to the plan, as the notes themselves should correspond to one or more objectives within the plan.

Benefits of utilizing the plan this way are multiple. First, it is a transparent and accessible way of working; all members of the team (including the person receiving services) are aware of their roles and others' roles in making progress toward the identified goals. For the practitioner, the requirements of documentation include charting directly to the stated goals and objectives. This is for several reasons, including making sure that the services provided are appropriate and billable (when relevant).

Importance of Progress Notes

- To record what was done, by whom, when, and with what effects.
- To describe significant changes in the person's status.
- To evaluate progress in relation to the goals and objectives on the care plan.
- To record consultations with other providers or natural supports.
- To facilitate communication and coordination.
- To provide a record of the person's recovery journey.
- To serve as a supervisory tool; supervisors use progress notes to see what you have been doing.

Progress notes are about evaluating the impact of the services provided within the context of the person's care plan. In this sense, they represent an important opportunity to reflect on whether or not the plan, as written, is helping the person to achieve his or her objectives and move closer to his or her recovery goals. If notes routinely reflect that a person is not making progress, it can be an indication that a roadblock has been encountered and a mid-course correction is needed. Finally, progress notes also work to ensure there is accountability among all stakeholders who have committed action steps to the plan, including the person in recovery and his or her natural supports. This is critical, as even the very best person-centered plan is only as good as its implementation and follow-through!

Essential Elements of a Progress Note

Specific pieces of information are key to include in any progress note. These vary by organization and funder, but generally must include, at a minimum:

- Name of person and other identifying information (e.g., medical record number)
- Date of service
- Location
- Time involved (including the duration of service as well as the specific time that services were delivered)
- What services were provided
- Signature, including discipline, and supervisor co-signature if required

Notes must accurately reflect the activity, location, and time for each service. The time indicated within the note includes the time spent in travel to deliver the service, plan progress review for the next steps, the actual provision of the service, and the documenting of the service.

As part of a person's medical, clinical, or health record, progress notes are considered legal documents. It is important that practitioners remain mindful of this status as they document their work and its impact. In addition to meetings with service users, practitioners need to document non-routine calls, missed sessions, and consultations with other professionals. Throughout, though, make sure that the focus is on the work being done and the person being served. Chart the person's successes as well as any significant concerns you may have, particularly if the person is disconnecting from care and you have concerns regarding his or her welfare. Given that progress notes and the chart as a whole are a legal document, remember that these can be subpoenaed at any time.

Types of Progress Notes

You may have a note writing system that is prescribed by your agency. The following are several examples of structuring the progress note itself into key elements. Each has an acronym that represents the different content areas of the note.

Elements of a DAP Note

Description: service delivered, impression of person, significant events, and status.

Analysis/Assessment: progress toward goals/objectives/interventions on the plan, person's response, and staff strategies.

Plan: the next contact, staff task, person in recovery task, or natural supporter task.

The DAP (Description, Analysis, and Plan) note starts with a description of the important information observed along with interventions, followed by an assessment of the person and of his or her response to the interventions, and concluding with a plan for the next steps, including the staff's next step, date of next contact, and any tasks for the person receiving services and his or her natural supporters.

Elements of a SOAP Note

Subjective: what the service-user states.

Objective: what you observed.

Assessment: description of the person's behavior/movement toward goals—not necessarily CLINICAL assessment.

Plan: the next contact, staff tasks, and person's tasks.

A second format for the progress note is that of SOAP. SOAP notes start with the "subjective," which includes what was said by the person receiving services, followed by "objective," or what you observed as the practitioner. Next, similar to the DAP note, is the "assessment": this is a description of the person's response and any progress following the intervention, including specifically addressing the movement toward objectives and goals. This note also ends with the plan for the future, including the staff's next step, date of next contact, and any tasks for the person receiving services and his or her natural supporters.

A third kind of progress note structure is the GIRPS (Goal, Intervention, Response, and Significant Observations). This is probably the most useful structure for writing billable progress notes for person-centered care approaches, as it includes the Goal and Objective aspect in the structure of the note. Continuously reflecting on these aspects of the plan serves as an important reminder of the person's most valued recovery goal, and keeps the team collectively focused on working together to help them move forward toward this destination.

Elements of a GIRPS Progress Note

Goal: related goal(s) and objective(s) from the plan.

Intervention: a description of the specific activities performed by the staff.

Response: person/family response to the above specific intervention; encourage inclusion of person/family self-assessment of response as well as staff assessment.

Plan for the next steps within the context of interventions and response.

Significant Observations: description of the person's presentation that is different from usual presentation including any recent or current circumstances that need to be taken into consideration.

An organization may decide to use any of these structures to document the work and progress being made with a person in recovery. Regardless of what structure is utilized, it is important to include aspects of culture and context within the content of the note, as discussed in the next section.

Maintaining the Person-Centered Dimension of Progress Notes

When writing notes, technical elements are essential to include in addition to following whatever structure or format your agency or organization has decided to use. At the same time, the content of the note should not be overshadowed by the structure and technical detail. Without minimizing these aspects (as they are key to quality plan implementation as well as the billing and payment for services), we need to consider the language and other elements that should be considered in writing the note.

In terms of language, for example, as much of the progress note as possible should be written in everyday language so that the person receiving the services would be able to understand what has been recorded. Especially when concurrent documentation is being used (see below), it will be important for service users to review what is being recorded in their health record and be given an opportunity to provide their input on the content. Even when this is not the case, the language used in progress notes should mirror as much as possible the language used in the PCCP, which, as we suggested in Module 2, should be accessible to the person and his or her natural supporters.

We are not suggesting that diagnostic and clinical terms can never be used, however. What we are suggesting is that when it is necessary to use such terms, they should be accompanied by a description in everyday language of how what they are referring to is seen or experienced in the person's everyday life. A common example of this would be describing the clinical phenomenon of "auditory hallucinations" as hearing the voices of significant figures in the person's life, which may be either harsh and critical or supportive and helpful (or a combination of both). Other examples include describing "thought disorder" or "cognitive disruptions" as having difficulty keeping thoughts together or having difficulties with concentration, memory, or following the thread of a conversation. Similarly, "hypomania" can be described as increases in activity rates or levels, "dysthymia" as sadness, and "mood lability" as unexpected changes in the person's moods over time. When framed in these ways, persons being served can learn to identify their difficulties, and signs of progress, taking on a more active and collaborative role in their own care.

Just as in the strength-based assessment and plan development, it is also important to consider cultural elements when composing progress notes. As every interaction represented the convergence of multiple cultures (e.g., the practitioner's cultural identity and background, the service user's cultural identity and background, the culture of the health care system), it is important as a practitioner to reflect these forces within the documentation of the note. This can include recording particular preferences and observations that are related directly to culture and referring to a person's background and worldview and how these impact your assessment, interventions, and plan. Cultural factors should be considered along with the person's own understanding of his or her situation and needs, especially to avoid viewing culturally influenced interpretations of these experiences as pathological. Seeing or hearing the voice of a deceased relative, for example, is considered a normal part of the grieving process in many cultures and does not always indicate the presence of hallucinations, which is understood as symptoms of an underlying illness. Important in this process is to be reflective about one's own biases and to be aware of potential personal pitfalls.

Concurrent Documentation

One approach to writing progress notes that was designed to increase efficiency, but which can also promote person-centered care, is writing it concurrently. This means writing the note while the person is actually meeting with you and having him or her review it (and perhaps even include his or her input). Doing so ensures transparency of the process and efficiency in terms of not having to wait until the person leaves to complete your documentation. Some of the benefits of concurrent documentation include[1]:

- Staff satisfaction—Staff are often weary of paperwork, especially when it seems to limit the amount of time that can be spent providing direct care. Engaging in concurrent documentation can free up valuable time to provide services and complete other requirements for staff, including supervision and consultation.
- Compliance with submission and billing requirements.
- Supports recovery-focused services through service user participation and benefit. The philosophy of recovery-oriented care also consists of increasing the transparency and including the person receiving services in as many aspects of care as possible. Inclusion in the process of documentation serves as a way of demystifying the process and furthers a sense of partnership.
- Empowers the person and family to be aware of and to influence the course of clinical assessment and interventions by providing a built-in point of shared reflection regarding the progress or lack of progress toward recovery goals. It involves the person in the recording of what happened, and can significantly improve communication by more quickly addressing misunderstandings or clarifying miscommunications.
- Increases person and family "buy-in" to care through real time feedback. The consistent and regular checking in with a person receiving services, or his or her loved ones, regarding their perceptions of progress can provide yet another point of engagement and alliance building in doing this collaborative work.
- Significant positive impact on engagement in services and rates of medication adherence [1]. A recent study with 10 CMHCs across the country examined the impact of person-centered planning training when combined with concurrent documentation. When compared to a control group providing standard care, the PCP and concurrent documentation intervention were associated with significantly greater engagement in services (as measure by decreases in appointment "no shows) and higher rates of medication adherence (as measured by clinician assessment and informed by self-report). Perhaps due to the increased "buy-in" referred to above, these study findings suggest that when individuals have greater control over their treatment through the creation of a person-centered plan that is squarely focused on their personal goals, they are more likely to actively participate in the therapeutic process and to take advantage of the recovery tools being offered to them.

Concurrent documentation should not interfere with the collaborative nature of the work being done with the person receiving services. Using concurrent documentation means

---

[1] The benefits are listed on the basis of the details from www.thenationalcouncil.org/galleries/resources-services%20files/Concurrent%20Documentation%20Slides%20Webinar%209-10-07.pdf

being systematic and well-planned about the time spent together in order to allow time to conduct concurrent documentation in collaboration with the person "not to interrupt a session, but as a collaborative effort between provider and client at the end of a session."[2]

When to Review the Plan

To keep the plan an active and "living" document, useful in the everyday provision of services and working toward goals, it is important to update the plan regularly and as necessary. Typically, plans are required by regulators to reassess quarterly—every 90 days—and this is the national standard as well. A plan that is built on 90-day increments demonstrates belief in change as it communicates a hopeful expectation of progress and movement within a relatively short time frame.

Reviewing the plan is also key to evaluate the effectiveness of the interventions being provided at each meeting and subsequently to determine whether or not the plan itself needs to be revised. This is especially important if a new intervention is to be determined as needed. It also is the case that in order to bill for interventions, they need to be indicated on the plan. Therefore, as soon as possible, the plan should be revised to include new interventions and this, too, should be done as much as possible in consultation with the person receiving services.

Objectives may need to be revised if you realize that you and/or the person you are working with have been too ambitious and have bitten off more than what you can chew. An example would be a person who is interested in going back to college has set as an objective to "complete one college class with a grade of at least a 'B' in the next 90 days." If in 3 weeks' time, the person has yet to enroll or even pick up the phone to make a call to the registrar's office, the goal will be too much of a step to start out with. This does not mean that the goal is unobtainable, but instead that you are presented with a chance to reevaluate the relative "size" of the objective with regard to where the person is now in his or her recovery. PCCPs should be designed as much as possible to build on successes; to do so, it is important to balance the high expectations of a recovery-oriented system (and of service users and families) with a realistic assessment of where the person is in his or her recovery at any given time, along with the resources he or she has at his or her disposal. It is possible, for example, that the person did not call the registrar because he or she cannot afford to enroll at that time. So when agreed-upon objectives appear to be out of reach, it may require both the practitioner and the person to scale back to more incremental steps that are achievable within the designated time frame. As described in Module 6, breaking long-term goals down into achievable, shorter-term objectives requires clinical skill and resourcefulness; the same is true of breaking ambitious objectives down into the intervening steps that need to be taken to get there.

Another possibility for the plan update is to consider adding or removing interventions as necessary and as the person's condition evolves. To continue the above example regarding someone interested in returning to college, if the original set of interventions had not included a supported education component, it could be added to the plan so that a supported education counselor could support the person in making the transition into taking first a college class after a lengthy absence from academics.

---

[2] www.omh.state.ny.us/omhweb/clinic_standards/faq.html

The input of the person being served is essential in person-centered plan updates, just as it is in the initial development of the plan. When rewriting and reevaluating the plan on an interim basis (revisions between the full plan review), it is useful, as much as possible, to include natural supports and family members as desired by the service user. This may not be possible in all circumstances, but is something to work toward whenever possible. Finally, remember that reviews of the plan should not be triggered only by crisis events. In a recovery-oriented planning process, it is equally important to be future-focused and goal-oriented. Therefore, the team should reconvene around events of success/accomplishment as well as crises to revisit care plans and discuss next steps.

What we have described thus far is how an individual's plan is to be reviewed and revised on an ongoing basis as his or her recovery unfolds over time. A parallel process can also take place at the agency or organizational level, as the process of care planning can itself become the object of review and revision as one focus of continuous quality improvement (CQI). It is to this topic that we turn next.

The Role of Continuous Quality Improvement

No matter how faithfully you follow the suggestions and practices outlined in this manual, your process for PCCP, implementation, and review will not be perfect. Fundamentally a human process, care planning and delivery are just as fallible, or imperfect, as the people performing them. In recognition of this fact, and in pursuit of a way to continuously improve the quality of the care offered, practitioners have developed strategies for the ongoing review and revision of care processes. The structure and strategies for identifying areas for improvement, making such improvements, and then evaluating whether or not the improvements accomplished what they set out to do is often referred to as CQI. The various processes involved in PCCP, implementation, and review can and should become the object of an agency or organization's CQI efforts.

> *Q*uality improvement is achieved by setting goals and objectives, developing performance indicators to measure the objectives, and collecting diverse data on system performance.
>
> —California Mental Health Planning Council, Partnerships for Quality [3]

It is important at the outset to point out that CQI is not an attempt to weed out or punish "bad apples." Instead, the principles of CQI rest on the philosophy that difficulties in performance are most often due to inadequate job structures, training offerings, or supervision and monitoring efforts, and that these aspects can always be changed to move toward improving performance [2].

In order to identify and rectify these barriers to quality performance, input should be sought from all of the relevant parties involved. As in any collaboration, each stakeholder in PCCP, including service users, family and other team members, practitioners, and administrators, has a unique perspective and set of skills to contribute to the overall quality improvement process.

Oftentimes, in practice, organizational quality improvement efforts are limited to the assessment of quality in the *process* of planning and delivering care. But limiting one's focus to these processes alone ignores the very reasons for which these processes were undertaken to begin with, that is, to achieve better *outcomes*. Remember the fourth and final "P" of person-centered planning discussed in Module 1. This refers to the importance of focusing on the ultimate expected *Product* of person-centered planning, with that product being the attainment of recovery and community inclusion outcomes deemed meaningful by service users and their loved ones. It is not enough simply to offer high quality clinical and rehabilitative services and supports if they do not achieve the outcomes for which they were designed. Rather, services and supports are means to an end, the end being the meaningful life in the community to which the service user and his or loved ones aspire. This section, therefore, addresses CQI as it relates both to *process* and *outcome* dimensions.

What Is the Role of the Supervisor in Promoting Quality and Accountability?

Supervisors are increasingly recognized as having a critical role to play in promoting CQI efforts in the area of person-centered care and planning. Supervisors are often in the unique and sometimes challenging position between administrators and direct care staff. Clear expectations of supervisors can help them to *lead by example*, to *set a positive tone* regarding the need for and benefit of CQI efforts, and therefore to do a better job supporting all stakeholders in the CQI process. These expectations include:

- Supervisors *set and communicate expectations* for staff performance through coaching staff in small groups, holding individual coaching sessions, and through in vivo, live coaching of person-centered interactions.
- Supervisors *monitor* staff performance on a regular and systematic basis, including review and feedback on plans as well as supervision on PCCP process.
- Supervisors compare staff performance and *recognize exemplary and improving PCCP practices.*
- Supervisors compare staff performance to established benchmark expectations and *identify priorities for needed improvements.*
- Supervisors *partner with others* in setting performance indicators for collaboration. Particularly crucial in this regard are supervisors' efforts to invite service users as well as family members to the table to define valued process indicators; for example, "I know my provider is supporting my wishes, hopes, and desires when … "
- Supervisors *provide information and data* to decision makers to guide program improvement and sustainability.
- Supervisors *provide coaching* to enhance staff's performance in CQI activities and target areas. Coaching can take multiple formats including:
  1. *Group coaching.* In this model, a supervisor uses a 15- to 60-min time period to help the entire staff brush up on their skills. Group coaching takes many forms, but often

uses role-play as a learning format. Role-play is often the best way to create cognitive dissonance in the learner's mind, which leads to new learning.

2. *One-on-one or paired coaching.* In this model, the supervisor works one-on-one with a staff person, or uses pairs of staff to set up mutual support for learning new skills.

3. *In vivo or live coaching.* In this model, the supervisor accompanies the staff and coaches live. The supervisor may step into the live interaction and model the skill, or may silently observe the skill being performed and later comment on it.

Through continual expectation setting, assessment, feedback, and coaching, supervisors can make a significant difference in the quality and delivery of PCCP. Supervisory support is but one piece of the puzzle making up quality improvement activities. The following section outlines the role of the service user in promoting quality as well.

What Is the Role of the Person in Recovery in Promoting Quality?

People who use services from an agency are vital members of the CQI team. Making sure that their involvement is meaningful, though, is key. Indicators of meaningful service user and family involvement include the following.

- People in recovery comprise a significant proportion of representatives to an agency's board of directors, advisory board, or other steering committees and work groups.
- People in recovery and their family members or loved ones are routinely invited to evaluate the quality of, and their satisfaction with, the services that are offered.
- Formal grievance procedures are established and made readily available to people in recovery and their family members to address dissatisfaction with services. These grievances are resolved in a way that supports and involves the affected person. Grievances are made transparent, that is, de-identified and shared widely across systems in aggregated ways, so as to educate all stakeholders about the issues that are being raised and the agency's attempts to respond.
- People are not penalized, denied services, or otherwise ostracized for exercising these rights to grieve or provide feedback in other ways.

Often, agencies may want to include family and service users, but find that they are not sure about how to do so. Table 7.1 outlines a few suggestions on how to promote meaningful participation in CQI efforts. Also provided at the conclusion of this module is an agency self-assessment of the various ways in which service users and family members or loved ones can be involved in an agency's efforts to monitor and improve the quality of the care offered, including its fidelity to the person-centered practices described in this manual. Developed as part of a Consumer, Youth, and Family Quality Improvement Collaborative funded by the State of Connecticut's Department of Mental Health and Addiction Services, this survey was structured to be administered by service users and family members themselves, in the hope that peer-to-peer administration would yield the most honest and accurate responses.

Table 7.1   Tips on Promoting Meaningful Involvement of Service Users and Families

- *Compensation*. Compensation for people's time and expenses can be a way both to promote involvement and to communicate a strong message that the value of their contributions is an essential piece of the agency's commitment to a service user and family-directed system.
- *Understanding Barriers*. Understand that the answer "not interested" from service users can have a wide range of reasons behind it. Ask people why they prefer NOT to be involved, and then address the barriers identified. For example, people may have little faith that their voice will be respected and acted on and it may take time for them to develop confidence in the process.
- *Not Just a Token*. Engaging more than one person in recovery in the process is important—it helps avoid the sense of tokenism and brings a stronger and more diverse set of voices to the table.
- *Peers Engaging Peers*. This is a particularly useful method for encouraging the active involvement of service users and families. Advocacy communities and peer programs can provide a great service by working on capacity building among persons in recovery and their loved ones to encourage and prepare them to be active agents in the CQI process.
- *Training and Education*. Leadership academies can support people to develop skills that allow them to be confident, vocal, and effective contributors to evaluation and quality processes.

Types of Continuous Quality Improvement

Process evaluation: monitoring the quality of plan development and implementation

The following are essential points to keep in mind as you work with the person and his or her recovery support network to monitor the quality of the PCCP *process*.

- Evaluation in a service user or family-directed paradigm is a continuous process, and expectations are high for successful outcomes in a broad range of quality-of-life dimensions (in areas such as employment, social connections, community membership). For example, many individuals express that the maintenance of "clinical stability" alone is not sufficient as a treatment outcome, as the experience of recovery is about much more than the absence of symptoms or distress.
- All major stakeholders involved in the PCCP process must have their input on evaluating the work of the team and the process of plan development.
- The individual using or receiving services drives the process and continues to have the lead role in the plan and evaluation of the process behind its development.
- Flexibility and responsibility to change course when necessary are essential.
- The ability to measure success (and incremental improvements in process and outcomes variables) must start with a meaningful benchmarking to determine where you are starting from and to plan for the road ahead.
- Clinical records and care plans, as well as service user feedback on the PCCP process, should be regularly reviewed by supervisors or quality assurance personnel to guarantee

conformance with the principles and practices of PCCP. The "proof is in the pudding" concept applies here. The delivery of person-centered care and care planning should be evidenced in the clinical record and confirmed by the direct solicitation of service users' and families' experiences.

Rating scales can be essential tools in data gathering. At the conclusion of this module, we provide several versions of one such data-gathering tool, the *Person-Centered Care Questionnaire* (PCCQ) [4]. This is a 32-item questionnaire that was developed specifically for work with individuals with mental health conditions to assess numerous process indicators of PCCP. Instrument data sources form the self-report of an individual's firsthand experience of the planning process, with parallel versions for practitioner self-assessment of behaviors and attitudes involved in PCCP and family members' self-report of their experiences as participants in the PCCP process.

In addition to using tools that assess adherence to PCCP best practices, it is useful to evaluate the overall quality of the "recovery environment" within which this planning is conducted. The *Compendium of Recovery Measures* [5] is an excellent resource for measurement strategies. A sample of one of the measures reviewed in this *Compendium*, the *Recovery Self-Assessment Scale* [6] is also available at the conclusion of this module for the readers' reference. More recent reviews of recovery-oriented measures have been completed by Burgess and colleagues [7] and Williams and colleagues [8].

Outcomes evaluation: Monitoring the impact of PCCP

As we noted above, the assessment of quality should not end with the rating of services or supports in a process evaluation. Though this is one important component in a coordinated CQI effort, it must be accompanied by simultaneous efforts to evaluate the impact of those services or supports on the lives of people in recovery and their loved ones through outcome evaluation. The plan itself is only a means to an end, and it is equally important to assess the degree to which improvements in performance lead to improvements in meaningful outcomes.

PCCP puts the focus on the person and his or her future, rather than on a set of services, programs, or treatments that can be offered to meet various needs and goals. The plan itself is not the goal, even if it is multifaceted, culturally relevant, and directed by the person or family. Rather, the plan is simply one pathway to a life complete with respect from others, meaningful opportunities and choices, personal responsibility, community/school presence and participation, and self-chosen supports [9].

For an extensive review of person-directed quality indicators that can be used in PCCP outcome evaluations, the reader is referred to the website of the Council on Quality and Leadership (CQL) at www.thecouncil.org/resources/. CQL provides training, technical assistance, and resource development to human service organizations nationally and internationally with a specific focus on teaching customers to become even better at ensuring that people with disabilities lead lives of dignity and quality. CQL's website offers a number of excellent, downloadable resources that can assist agencies in carrying out both process and outcome evaluations as a means of improving overall quality. One example of CQL's approach to measuring quality is their Personal Outcomes Measure [10] that provides a powerful data set for the valid and reliable measurement of individual quality of life. Instead of looking at the quality of how the services are being delivered, the Personal Outcome Measures approach looks at whether the services and supports have the desired results or outcomes that matter to the individual.

While the CQL is perhaps best known for its contributions toward promoting person-centered process and outcomes in support of persons with developmental and/or physical disabilities, its tools hold equal relevance for persons living with *psychiatric* disabilities given their focus not on the individual's label or diagnosis but on the shared outcomes that are often common aspirations of ALL human beings. For readers who are interested in the application of recovery-based outcomes measures designed specifically for use with individuals living with mental health conditions, the following are user-friendly and brief instruments the authors have used in numerous research and evaluation efforts to assess outcomes likely to be impacted by the implementation of Person-Centered Care Planning: The Recovery Markers Questionnaire [11], the Brief Recovery Assessment Scale [12], the Empowerment Scale [13], and the Herth Hope Index [14].

Practitioner Self-Evaluation

Now that you know the various components of, and the processes involved in, PCCP, how will you know when you are implementing these well in practice? This concluding section offers questions for practitioner self-reflection to assess your own progress in developing and implementing PCCPs. In addition to the tools referenced earlier in this module, for example, the PCCQ (Provider Version), Table 7.2 summarizes the eight primary questions that you can use to assess your own care plans in terms of their person-centeredness. We then describe each of these dimensions in more detail.

1. Does the PCCP appear to be specific to a unique individual, or could it equally be used for multiple clients as well? Is it based on an individual's personally defined life goals and informed by his or her personal needs, values, and preferences? PCCP can be carried out

Table 7.2   Questions for Self-Assessment of Person-Centered Care Planning

Does the Person-Centered Care Plan	Yes	No
1. Appear to be specific to a unique individual?		
2. Provide you and your client with a roadmap?		
3. Base interventions and actions steps on the client's personal strengths and interests?		
4. Address what the client will be doing between appointments?		
5. Clearly delineate the tasks and roles to be performed?		
6. Change over time?		
7. Encourage and support the client in assuming increasing control over his or her life?		
8. Contain language that is accessible and understandable?		

only at the level of each individual person within the context of his or her family and life. Each client's PCCP should thus look different from everyone else's and be based squarely on his or her own particular history, experiences, challenges, and perspective.

2. Does the PCCP provide you and your client with a roadmap for where you are headed together and what he or she is trying to do in his or her life? Does the plan envision a life outside of or beyond formal mental health services, or does it remain within the boundaries of the mental health system? Can you tell from the plan what the care team and the client are trying to accomplish (e.g., education, a job, increased independence, more friends), not just what you are trying to get rid of or avoid (e.g., symptoms, substance use)? If medication is part of the plan, can you say what the medication is to be used for? How will you know when it is working or not working? Is adherence to treatment viewed as an end in itself, or is it viewed as a route to some other, personally desirable end? Will the services offered lead the client toward some worthwhile and wished for changes in his or her life?

3. Does the PCCP base interventions and action steps on the client's personal strengths and interests, or are they based entirely on his or her diagnoses and problems? Is it clear how the care team will help the client to identity and utilize his or her strengths, both their own and those within their social environment? Can you say from the plan what the client's specific interests are, and how these interests have contributed to the formulation of goals and objectives? Does the plan help the client to move toward what interests him or her, or does it simply try to move him or her away from problematic behaviors or activities? If substance abuse is identified as a problem to be addressed, for example, does the plan also address what kind of sober activities the client may want to participate in instead? Are community activities and resources identified in the plan that would support the client in pursing his or her interests? Are there people identified in the plan with whom the client can share these interests?

4. Does the PCCP address what the client will be doing between mental health, and other health care, appointments? Does it outline more for the client to do than simply to receive treatment or attend meetings with practitioners? As treatment and rehabilitation are tools to be used by the client to reclaim a whole and gratifying life, it is essential for any interventions that are offered to be useful for these purposes. Does the client understand why he or she needs certain treatments, or why practitioners expect him or her to attend meetings or groups? Is it clear to the client how these activities will help him or her to get where he or she wants to in life, or do they simply seem to aim to keep the client busy? Does the care team take an interest in how the client spends his or her time between appointments? Does the plan include concrete suggestions for things the client might try in the community, and who he or she might try these activities with, or does the plan stipulate that the client is to participate only in mental health-related activities?

5. Does the PCCP clearly delineate the tasks and roles to be performed and the parties responsible for each? Does the plan clearly identify the client's own sphere of responsibility and the tasks that he or she has agreed to take on? Does the plan identify things the client can do to pursue recovery? Does the plan suggest how progress toward recovery is to be identified or assessed? Does the plan identify the next one or two steps in the client's recovery and sketch out, no matter how provisionally, what will be involved in his or her taking these next few steps? Does the plan include or suggest strategies for managing symptoms that do not go away in response to medication?

6. Does the PCCP, and the care provided based on it, change over time with the client's evolving goals and needs? PCCPs do not accept maintenance as a valid goal, as people do not want merely to be "maintained." It is quite possible for people to want to maintain a level of clinical stability, or to want to remain at a plateau of functioning for an extended period of time. Few people like change for the sake of change, and many people are afraid of taking risks or trying out new things because of a very legitimate fear that they might suffer a setback (a fear often reinforced by caring practitioners who do not want to see people relapse). But life does not stand still. Therefore, while avoiding symptoms or containing an illness or addiction may be a very real concern and goal for a given client at a given time, it is not possible to do so simply by "maintaining" one's current status that is, by trying to stand still. PCCPs thus anticipate that change is inevitable and that the client will need to continue to adapt to new situations and new challenges, whether he or she likes to or not. One important contribution recovery-oriented practices can make in such situations is to help the client identify those things that he or she wants to keep the same while other things around them are changing.

7. Does the PCCP encourage and support the client in assuming increasing control over his or her life, including the power to make his or her own decisions? Because of a history of paternalism and maternalism in psychiatry, the client may need to be encouraged to take back the control of certain parts of his or her life, the responsibility for which may have been assumed by other people. Does the plan encourage the client to do so? Does the plan remind the client of, or introduce him or her, to his or her strengths and gifts? Does the plan identify small successes, or easy wins, in order to help the client rebuild his or her self-confidence and sense of personal efficacy? Does the plan encourage and support the client in taking risks and trying new things—perhaps even prodding him or her gently to get unstuck, to be liberated from the inertia of a chronic illness?

8. Finally, is the language used in the PCCP accessible and understandable to the client and his or her supporters? Just as the plan needs to identify the client's role in promoting or pursuing his or her recovery, the plan and the care offered need to be accessible to and understandable by the client as well. Does the plan address those aspects of the client's own experiences that are of concern to him or her, and in a language that he or she will be able to understand and to use (e.g., voices as opposed to auditory hallucinations, feeling unsafe, vulnerable, or unprotected as opposed to paranoia)? Does the client know what care he or she has agreed to receive or participate in? Has his or her consent been truly informed, or are things done to the client that he or she has not agreed to? Even in cases in which the client is being treated involuntarily, or has a conservator or guardian assigned, have concerted efforts been made to inform the client of the available options and to explain what he or she can expect to happen, including what needs to happen for the client to no longer receive care involuntarily or no longer need a guardian or conservator?

Workforce Development as an Essential Part of Continuous Quality Improvement

For some practitioners, PCCP as presented through this manual may be highly consistent with current practice. For others, it may represent a significant shift—in which case it is critical also to discuss the corresponding shift in skills and competencies that are required in order to be an effective supporter of a quality PCCP process. In other words, what does a provider need to know to be able to offer recovery-oriented, person-centered care and planning?

Defining recovery competencies

The majority of efforts to date to define recovery competencies have focused on the identification of systems-level indicators rather than individual practitioner competencies. Some examples of systems-level indicators are reviewed in:

- *Characteristics of recovery-oriented mental health programs: Can I recognize one if I see one?* [15].
- National Technical Assistance Center's landmark report: *Mental Health Recovery: What Helps and What Hinders* [16].
- *Recovery as policy in mental health services: Strategies emerging from the states* [17].

These types of efforts have made significant contributions to advancing the field's knowledge and understanding recovery-enhancing environments.

An example of efforts to define individual *practitioner level competencies* can be found in the Los Angeles Mental Illness Research, Education, and Clinical Center (MIRECC) Competencies Initiative. This initiative involved the development of a set of core clinical competencies that support the goals of empowerment and rehabilitation among individuals with serious mental illnesses [18]. One product of the MIRECC initiative was the development of the CAI, the Competency Assessment Instrument [19], a measure that evaluates competencies viewed as central to recovery-oriented care. The CAI contains 55 items across 15 scales in a user-friendly format that can be applied to individuals or, collectively, to assess team-based competencies.

Other efforts to identify provider level competencies include international projects such as the *Recovery Competencies for New Zealand Mental Health Workers* [20] that details core recovery competencies in 10 different domains and provides corresponding resource lists to guide provider education and skill development. Similarly, the Center for Psychiatric Rehabilitation at Boston University, a national leader in research and training in recovery-oriented care, is in the process of examining this issue through an Internet Survey on Professional Practices that Promote Recovery. This survey of mental health service users and practitioners invites individuals to share their perspectives on how practitioners can facilitate and promote recovery from serious mental illness. For additional information, see www.bu.edu/cpr/recoverysurvey/.

Summary

In summary, documentation of progress notes and modifications to the plan should reflect the key principles of person-centered approaches, including striving to be transparent, inclusive, and collaborative, with a focus on the person's hopes and dreams. Documentation is a part of recording the journey and assessing progress on a regular basis. Doing so helps promote hope and allows the practitioner and the person receiving services to regularly reassess and change course when necessary in order to promote recovery.

The second half of this module emphasizes the need for practitioners and administrators to stimulate positive change and CQI by identifying and responding to key organizational context issues. It is equally important that the recovery community be organized and activated to demand necessary changes in systems of care so that they may promote person-centered care and care planning. For example, independent advocates can be trained and involved in planning sessions so that they can help ensure adherence to PCCP best practices. This highlights an important message on which to end this module:

> *Everyone has a role in recovery. Consumers and families must become informed and ask for what works … Policy people and administrators must read the research about effective services and they must examine laws, rules, and policies to root out discrepancies. They must be relentless in changing what does not support recovery. They must expect outcomes for public dollars. Direct service staff must cultivate their own personal characteristics that support recovery: creativity, flexibility, persistence, empathy, and the avoidance of objectifying people. They must know what supports outcomes and be willing to upgrade their skills when new techniques appear to be useful.*
>
> Selleck and colleagues [21]

Additional Tools and Resources

1. <u>Agency Self-Assessment on the Involvement of Service Users and Family Members/</u>
   <u>Significant Others in Quality Improvement Activities:</u>
   (Administrator & Staff Version) Developed by the Consumer, Youth, and
   Family Quality Improvement Collaborative of the State of Connecticut [22]

Rate, on a 1 to 5 scale, the degree to which this agency...	Not at all				Fully
1. Has established the involvement of service users and family members/significant others in quality improvement activities as a priority.	1	2	3	4	5
2. Frequently and regularly invites service users and family members/significant others to provide immediate feedback to practitioners regarding the quality and responsiveness of the care they receive.	1	2	3	4	5
3. Collects measures of service users and family members/significant others' satisfaction with care routinely and in a timely fashion.	1	2	3	4	5
4. Uses findings of service user and family member/significant other satisfaction surveys, as well as other input and feedback from them, to improve care.	1	2	3	4	5
5. Recruits a diverse group of service users and family members/significant others that are representative of the populations served to take part in both ongoing and focused quality improvement activities.	1	2	3	4	5
6. Adequately prepares service users and family members/significant others for their various roles in agency quality improvement activities.	1	2	3	4	5
7. Involves service users and family members/significant others in conducting needs assessments and in identifying priorities for resource allocation and service and support development.	1	2	3	4	5
8. Involves service users and family members/significant others in designing and developing new services and supports.	1	2	3	4	5
9. Involves service users and family members/significant others in establishing expectations for and outcomes of care.	1	2	3	4	5
10. Involves service users and family members/significant others in evaluating the effectiveness of care and efforts to promote wellness.	1	2	3	4	5
11. Values the contributions of service users and family members/significant others to quality improvement activities, as evidenced by providing feedback about changes made in response to their input and by reimbursing them commensurately for their time.	1	2	3	4	5
12. Has safeguards in place to ensure service users and family members/ significant others will not suffer retribution for offering their input.	1	2	3	4	5
13. Informs interested service users and family members/significant others of opportunities to participate in quality improvement activities at the level of the local, regional, or statewide system.	1	2	3	4	5

2. <u>Survey on the Involvement of Service Users and Family Members in Mental Health Quality Improvement Activities:</u> **(Service User version)** Developed by the Consumer, Youth, and Family Quality Improvement Collaborative of the State of Connecticut [22]

Introduction for Service Users:

Hi. My name is _____. I receive mental health services myself/ have a family member who receives mental health services and I am an advocate trying to improve the quality of the mental health care people receive in _____. I am excited to visit with you today to get a sense of what your experiences have been like as a user of mental health services in _____. There will be no right or wrong answers to these questions. They only ask about your own experiences. And no one will know how you answered these questions, since you will not put your name on the form. Your answers will be kept confidential from the staff here and at all other mental health agencies. I think this interview will take about 15 minutes, and if there is any statement you do not understand or are not sure how to answer, just let me know.

I am also very interested in any experiences you may have had in trying to improve the quality of the care you, or others, receive from mental health agencies and organizations in _____. So some of these questions will ask more broadly about your participation in these kinds of activities, but we will get to those in a few minutes. For now, let's focus on your own care.

Town Where Services are

Received:_____

Age: _____   **Gender:** _____   **Years receiving care:** _____

Culture/race/ethnicity:_____

Please rate, on a scale from 5 to 1, how often you have had the following experiences:

Rate the statement a 5 if you have this experience all of the time, a 4 if you have it often, a 3 if you have it sometimes, a 2 if you have it seldom, and a 1 if you have never had it. If you don't know or are not sure, we can rate it a 0.	5	4	3	2	1	0
1. Providers explain what choices you have of services and supports available to you at their agency.						
2. Providers explain both the positives and negatives about the services and supports available to you.						
3. Providers explain services and supports available to you outside of their particular agency.						
4. Providers ask you about your own goals.						
5. You are involved in making decisions about your care.						
6. You participate in treatment team review or recovery planning meetings about your care.						
7. Providers ask if you need transportation or childcare to keep your appointments.						

	5	4	3	2	1	0
8. Providers encourage you to include family members, friends, and/or other people in your mental health care.						
9. Providers encourage you to tell them what you think about your care or when you want to change providers.						
10. You feel comfortable telling providers what you think about your care at any time.						
11. When you have expressed concerns about your care, you have received a respectful and timely response.						
12. Providers have told you how to go about filing a formal grievance if you have serious concerns about your care.						
13. You feel confident that you will not suffer any consequences for offering your opinions or feedback about your care.						
14. Providers have asked you about your cultural background and how it might impact your care. (By culture we include race, ethnicity, gender, sexual preference, and religious affiliation).						
15. Providers are aware of and respect your cultural background and its importance to you.						
16. Providers have talked with you about writing a Psychiatric Advance Directive.						

Now I'd like to turn to those other questions I mentioned, that ask more about any experiences you may have had trying to improve the quality of mental health services. These usually fall under the umbrella of what is called "quality improvement," and there are a number of different activities that fall under this umbrella. These may include filling out satisfaction surveys, designing satisfaction surveys, conducting assessments, identifying priorities for how money is spent on services, developing new services, or helping to decide how services should be evaluated.

Again, there are no right or wrong answers to these questions. We are only interested in your own experiences. The scale is the same here, from 5 meaning all the time to 1 meaning never. And once again, if you don't know or are not sure, we can rate it a 0.

Please rate on a scale of 5 to 1, how often you have had the following experiences:

	5	4	3	2	1	0
Rate the statement a 5 if you have this experience all of the time, a 4 if you have it often, a 3 if you have it sometimes, a 2 if you have it often, and a 1 if you have never had it. If you do not know or if you are not sure that you have ever had this experience, we can rate it a 0.						
17. You have been invited to participate in some of these quality improvement activities I've just mentioned.						

18. Providers have asked you to rate your level of satisfaction with the care you receive.		
19. When you have been involved in quality improvement activities, your contributions have been taken seriously.		
20. When you have been involved in quality improvement activities, you have been paid for your time.		

Is there anything else you would like us to know about your experience as a user of mental health services?

3. <u>Person-Centered Care Questionnaire</u> (Provider Version and Person in Recovery Version. Note: Contact authors for Administrator and Family Member/Significant Other Versions). Developed by Tondora & Miller, 2009 [4].

Person-Centered Care Planning Questionnaire
Provider Version
(Tondora & Miller, 2009)

Please indicate the degree to which you agree or disagree with the following statements about your approach to treatment or recovery planning.

1	2	3	4	5	DK
Strongly disagree	Somewhat disagree	Neither agree nor disagree	Somewhat agree	Strongly agree	Don't know

		1	2	3	4	5	DK
1.	I remind each person that she or he can bring family members or friends to recovery planning meetings.						
2.	I offer each person a copy of his or her plan to keep.						
3.	I write recovery goals in each person's own words.						
4.	Recovery plans are written so that each person and his or her family members can understand them. When professional language is necessary, I explain it.						
5.	I ask each person to include healing practices in his or her plan that are based on his or her cultural background.						
6.	I encourage each person to include other providers, like vocational or housing specialists, in their meetings.						
7.	I include each person's strengths, interests, and talents in his or her plan.						
8.	I link each person's strengths to objectives in his or her plan.						
9.	I make sure that plans include the next few concrete steps that each person has greed to work on.						
10.	I include those areas of each person's life that he or she wants to work on (like health, social relationships, getting a job, housing, and spirituality) in his or her plan.						
11.	I try hard to understand how each person accounts for what has happened to them and how they see their experiences based on their cultural background.						
12.	I include in recovery plans the goals that each person tells me are important to them.						
13.	I develop care plans in a collaborative way with each person I serve.						
14.	I encourage each person to set the agenda for his or her recovery planning meetings.						
15.	I use "person-first" langauge when referring to people in the plan, (e.g., "a person with schizophrenia" rather than a "schizophrenic")						
16.	I consider cultural factors (such as the person's spiritual beliefs and culturally-based health/illness beliefs) in all parts of the recovery planning process						

17.	I let each person know ahead of time about their recovery planning meetings.						
18.	I include goals and objectives in recovery plans that address what each person want to get back in his or her life, not just what he or she is trying to avoid or get rid of.						
19.	I explain to each person how much time they have to work on each step in their plan.						
20.	As part of planning meetings, I educate each person about his or her rights and responsibilities in care.						
21.	I identify an explicit role and action step(s) for each person in the interventions section of his or her plan.						
22.	I also identify explicit roles/action steps for each person's supporters in the interventions section of the plan.						
23.	I offer education about personal wellness and self-determination tools such as WRAP and advance directives as part of the planning process.						
24.	The interventions and action steps identified in the plan encourage the person's connection to integrated/natural settings and supporters (rather than segregated settings designed only for people with mental illness).						
25.	I ask about cultural beliefs and areas of each person's cultural background that I do not understand to enhance the cultural relevance of the planning process.						
26.	I support people in pursuing goals such as housing or employment, even if they are still struggling actively with medication adherence, sobriety, or clinical symptoms.						
27.	I offer education about peer-based services and mutual support groups as part of the planning process.						
28.	If requested or needed, I utilize bilingual/bicultural translators throughout the care process.						
29.	I build attention to each person's cultural preferences and values into the process of writing a person-centered plan.						
30.	Each person is involved in the recovery planning process as much as he or she wants to be.						
31.	I identify the purpose of each intervention in the plan to link it to the person's identified goals and objectives.						
32.	I give each person the chance to review and make changes to his or her care plan.						

The best part of the recovery planning process has been..._____

_____

If I could change something about recovery planning, it would be... _____

_____

Person-Centered Care Planning Questionnaire
Person in Recovery (PIR) Version
(Tondora & Miller, 2009)

Please indicate the degree to which you agree or disagree with the following statements about your experiences of treatment or recovery planning.

1	2	3	4	5	DK
Strongly disagree	Somewhat disagree	Neither agree nor disagree	Somewhat agree	Strongly agree	Don't know

		1	2	3	4	5	DK
1.	My provider reminds me that I can bring my family, friends, or other supportive people to my recovery planning meetings.						
2.	I get a copy of the recovery plan to keep.						
3.	My goals are written in my own words in the plan.						
4.	My recovery plan is written so that I can understand it. Words that I don't understand are explained to me.						
5.	I was able to include healing practices based on my culture in the plan.						
6.	I can invite other providers, like my vocational or housing specialist, to the meeting if I want.						
7.	My strengths and talents are talked about in my plan.						
8.	In my plan, I can see how I'll use my strengths to work on my goals.						
9.	In my plan, there are next steps for me and my provider to work on.						
10.	Those areas of my life that I want to work on (like health, social relationships, getting a job, housing, and spirituality) are talked about and included in my plan if I want them.						
11.	My recovery team really understood how I explained what was going on for me, based on how I see it in my culture.						
12.	The goals in my plan are important to me.						
13.	I feel like when my provider and I work on a recovery plan, we work together as a team.						
14.	I decide how the meeting is run and what we'll talk about during my recovery planning meeting.						
15.	In my plan, my provider refers to me as "a person with" a mental health issue and does not define me by a label, e.g., "a schizophrenic" or "a bipolar."						
16.	Cultural factors (such as my spiritual beliefs and my cultural views) are considered in my plan.						
17.	I know ahead of time about when my recovery planning meeting is going to happen.						

		1	2	3	4	5	DK
18.	My plan talks about what I want to get back in my life, not just what I'm trying to get rid of.						
19.	I know what amount of time I have to work on each step in my plan.						
20.	As part of my planning meetings, I get education about my rights and about my responsibilities in treatment.						
21.	As part of the plan, I have things that I'm supposed to do to work on my goals.						
22.	Other people, like my friends and family, have things that they are supposed to do to help me work on my plan, and those things are written in the plan.						
23.	I am offered education about personal wellness, advanced directives, and Wellness Recovery Action Planning (WRAP) as part of my planning meeting.						
24.	I feel like my plan helps me get back involved in my community, not just in places that provide services for people with mental illness.						
25.	My provider asked me about parts of my culture that she or he did not understand to make the recovery plan better for me.						
26.	I feel like my provider supports me in working on things like getting a job and managing my money, even if I still have other issues.						
27.	I got information about peer support as part of my planning meeting.						
28.	If needed, I was able to get a bilingual/bicultural translator for my recovery planning meeting.						
29.	I feel like my culture was really taken into consideration when working on my recovery plan.						
30.	I feel involved in the recovery planning process.						
31.	It is clear to me in my plan how certain interventions/treatments will help me achieve my goals.						
32.	I have the chance to review and make changes to my plan.						

The best part of the recovery planning process has been..._____

_____

_____

If I could change something about recovery planning, it would be...

_____

_____

_____

4. Recovery-Self-Assessment-Revised. (Provider Version only. Note: Contact authors for Administrator, Person in Recovery, and Family Member/Significant Other Versions). Developed by O'Connell *et al.*, 2005 [6].

Recovery Self-Assessment-Revised

Provider Version
(O'Connell, et al., 2005)

Please circle the number below which reflects how accurately the following statements describe the activities, values, policies, and practices of this program.

1	2	3	4	5
Strongly Disagree				Strongly Agree

N/A= Not Applicable
D/K= Don't Know

1. Staff make a concerted effort to welcome people in recovery and help them to feel comfortable in this program.   1 2 3 4 5 N/A D/K

2. This program/agency offers an inviting and dignified physical environment (e.g., the lobby, waiting rooms, etc.).   1 2 3 4 5 N/A D/K

3. Staff encourage program participants to have hope and high expectations for their recovery.   1 2 3 4 5 N/A D/K

4. Program participants can change their clinician or case manager if they wish.   1 2 3 4 5 N/A D/K

5. Program participants can easily access their treatment records if they wish.   1 2 3 4 5 N/A D/K

6. Staff do not use threats, bribes, or other forms of pressure to influence the behavior of program participants.   1 2 3 4 5 N/A D/K

7. Staff believe in the ability of program participants to recover.   1 2 3 4 5 N/A D/K

8. Staff believe that program participants have the ability to manage their own symptoms.   1 2 3 4 5 N/A D/K

9. Staff believe that program participants can make their own life choices regarding things such as where to live, when to work, whom to be friends with, etc.   1 2 3 4 5 N/A D/K

10. Staff listen to and respect the decisions that program participants make about their treatment and care.   1 2 3 4 5 N/A D/K

11. Staff regularly ask program participants about their interests and the things they would like to do in the community.   1 2 3 4 5 N/A D/K

12. Staff encourage program participants to take risks and try new things.   1 2 3 4 5 N/A D/K

13. This program offers specific services that fit each participant's unique culture and life experiences.   1 2 3 4 5 N/A D/K

14. Staff offer participants opportunities to discuss their spiritual needs and interests when they wish.   1 2 3 4 5 N/A D/K

15. Staff offer participants opportunities to discuss their sexual needs and interests when they wish.   1 2 3 4 5 N/A D/K

16. Staff help program participants to develop and plan for life goals beyond managing symptoms or staying stable (e.g., employment, education, physical fitness, connecting with family and friends, hobbies).   1 2 3 4 5 N/A D/K

17. Staff routinely assist program participants with getting jobs.   1 2 3 4 5 N/A D/K

18. Staff actively help program participants to get involved in non-mental health/addiction related activities, such as church groups, adult education, sports, or hobbies.   1 2 3 4 5 N/A D/K

19. Staff work hard to help program participants to include people who are important to them in their recovery/treatment planning (such as family, friends, clergy, or an employer).   1 2 3 4 5 N/A D/K

20. Staff actively introduce program participants to persons in recovery who can serve as role models or mentors.   1 2 3 4 5 N/A D/K

21. Staff actively connect program participants with self-help, peer support, or consumer advocacy groups and programs.   1 2 3 4 5 N/A D/K

22. Staff actively help people find ways to give back to their community (i.e., volunteering, community services, neighborhood watch/cleanup).   1 2 3 4 5 N/A D/K

23. People in recovery are encouraged to help staff with the development of new groups, programs, or services.   1 2 3 4 5 N/A D/K

24. People in recovery are encouraged to be involved in the evaluation of this agency's programs, services, and service providers.   1 2 3 4 5 N/A D/K

25. People in recovery are encouraged to attend agency advisory boards and management meetings.   1 2 3 4 5 N/A D/K

26. Staff talk with program participants about what it takes to complete or exit the program.   1 2 3 4 5 N/A D/K

27. Progress made towards an individual's own personal goals is tracked regularly.   1 2 3 4 5 N/A D/K

28. The primary role of agency staff is to assist a person with fulfilling his/her own goals and aspirations.   1 2 3 4 5 N/A D/K

29. Persons in recovery are involved with facilitating staff trainings and education at this program.   1 2 3 4 5 N/A D/K

30. Staff at this program regularly attend trainings on cultural competency.   1 2 3 4 5 N/A D/K

31. Staff are knowledgeable about special interest groups and activities in the community.   1 2 3 4 5 N/A D/K

32. Agency staff are diverse in terms of culture, ethnicity, lifestyle, and interests.   1 2 3 4 5 N/A D/K

Exercises

Exercise 1. Evaluating Quality Elements in Progress Notes

Review the sample progress notes below which chart to Mr. Blake's person-centered Recovery Plan presented at the consultation of Module 6. Using some of the progress note structures presented earlier in this module (i.e., DAP, SOAP, GIRPS), evaluate each note for the required elements. Consider how these sample notes compare with the structure and content of progress notes you currently writing.

SAMPLE PROGRESS NOTES FOR MR. BLAKE
(REFER TO MODULE 6 FOR MR. BLAKE NARRATIVE AND PLAN)

Location: Community	x	Office		Type of Service: Ind			Group	X
Goal(s) Number:	1. *I want control of my money back.*		Objective(s) Number:		1. Budgeting monthly			
Present at Session ☒ Individual Present (If others, please identify name(s) and relationship(s) to individual):								
Interventions Provided (Please continue on back if necessary)	Demonstrated to Mr. Blake how to identify and list categories for types of expenses. Coached Mr. Blake in thinking through his monthly needs by talking through all of his expenditures from the last month. Provided Mr. Blake with a worksheet so that he can continue this work at home.							
Individual Response to the Intervention/ Plan and Next Steps	Mr. Blake was excited to get started on his budgeting, but had trouble concentrating and required redirection several times, as he easily became distracted by his strong feelings about not already being allowed to budget his money. He was able to refocus on the task, and was pleased that he was able to identify a number of his expenses in group, e.g., *"Pretty soon, I'll have enough saved for a security deposit on a new place!"* Mr. Blake agreed that he would work with his cousin over the next several days to more thoroughly identify his expenses. At our next session on 1/24/11 at 10:00 we will go over the worksheet that I gave him for homework.							
Signature and Credentials of Staff		Date of Signature	Date of Service	Start Time	Stop Time	Total Minutes		
Mary Tomason, BA		1/17/13	1/17/13	11:00	12:00	60		

Location: Community	X	Office		Type of Service: Ind	X		Group	
Goal(s) Number:	2. *I want to manage my meds on my own.*		Objective(s) Number:		1. Self-administering p.m. dose			
Present at Session ☒ Individual Present (If others, please identify name(s) and relationship(s) to individual):								
Interventions Provided (Please continue on back if necessary)	Met with Mr. Blake in his apartment to review his medication doses. Educated Mr. Blake about each pill, and coached Mr. Blake in making a list of his medications, including writing down the color and shape to aid with identification. Cued Mr. Blake on where to find dosage listings on his medication bottles as Mr. Blake could not initially do so on his own.							
Individual Response to the Intervention/ Plan and Next Steps	Mr. Blake was frustrated at first when going over his list of meds, stating that he *"already knew how to do this,"* although he was unable to make a list on his own at his first attempt. Upon completing his list, Mr. Blake expressed satisfaction and seemed proud to have his list, which he decided to post next to his calendar to make it accessible. Discussed with Mr. Blake that he would review his list with his visiting nurse to show his progress, and that we would plan on discussing strategies for afternoon reminders at our next visit.							
Signature and Credentials of Staff		Date of Signature	Date of Service	Start Time	Stop Time	Total Minutes		
Rashida Waters BA		1/18/13	1/18/13	1:15pm	1:45pm	30		
Location: Community		Office	X	Type of Service: Ind			Group	X
Goal(s) Number:	3. *I want to have friends and family in my life.*		Objective(s) Number:		1. Increasing social activities			
Present at Session ☒ Individual Present (If others, please identify name(s) and relationship(s) to individual):								
Interventions Provided (Please continue on back if necessary)	Mr. Blake was 10 minutes late to group and did not greet group members when he arrived. Prompted Mr. Blake to greet others. Led Mr. Blake through a role-play on meeting a new person in a community setting. Provided coaching to Mr. Blake on making small talk about the weather.							
Individual Response to the Intervention/ Plan and Next Steps	Mr. Blake was initially reluctant to participate in a role-play, but with encouragement from his fellow group members he did so. He needed specific cueing around asking questions to start conversations, but was able to independently and successfully end the role-played conversation. He had very good eye contact and he was open to the positive feedback from other members, e.g., *"I hear you. Sometimes I ramble and don't let folks get a word in edgewise."* For next steps, Mr. Blake could use further assistance with greeting others when he arrives into new situations. We will practice this at our next session on 1/26 at 12:15.							
Signature and Credentials of Staff		Date of Signature	Date of Service	Start Time	Stop Time	Total Minutes		
Jerry Angelus BA		1/19/13	1/19/13	12:15	1:15	60		

Exercise 2. Key Indicators in PCCP: You'll Know You're Doing it When ...

Part A: Complete the Provider Version of the Person-Centered Care Planning Questionnaire presented earlier in this module using your current practices to guide your answers. Then, consider the questions which follow.

1. Based on filling out this questionnaire about PCCP, what key areas of process or practice do you feel you need further clarification on?
2. What things seem already to be strong in practice?
3. What key areas need the most attention? How might these areas be strengthened?
4. What were you most surprised about in completing this exercise?

Part B: Invite at least one service user to complete the Person in Recovery Version of the Person-Centered Care Planning Questionnaire presented earlier in this module. Ask them to use their recent experiences in recovery planning with you to guide their answers. Encourage them to respond as openly as possible as the aim of this exercise is to garner their perspective on the quality of the process so that you can partner as effectively as possible in the co-creation of person-centered recovery plans. Following this exercise, discuss the following questions with the service user.

1. What were the service user's 3 highest and 3 lowest rated items?
2. Discuss how these responses compared to your own self-assessment completed in part A.
3. Is there anything NOT reflected in the PCCQ that is important to the service user in their experience of partnering with you in person-centered care planning?
4. What did you learn from "comparing notes" and how might this inform future improvements in both the process and documentation of person-centered care planning?

Learning Assessment

Module 7: Plan Implementation and Quality Monitoring		
Statement	True	False
1. Progress notes can be used as a supervisory tool.		
2. Concurrent documentation is a way of promoting empowerment and collaboration in the work with people receiving services.		
3. Culture does not need to be considered when documenting in progress notes.		
4. Progress notes chart directly to the goals, objectives, and interventions on the care plan.		
5. An essential feature of client satisfaction is agreement with staff on plan generation and development.		
See the Answer Key at the end of the chapter for the correct answers. Number Correct		
0 to 2: Don't be discouraged. Learning is an ongoing process! You can review the module for greater knowledge. 3 to 4: Great start. You can continue to use this guide to learn more about planning for recovery. 5: Nice! Use this guide to share what you've learned with others!		

References

1. Stanhope, V, Ingoglia, C, Schmelter, B *et al.* (2013). Impact of person-centered planning and collaborative documentation on treatment adherence. *Psychiatric Services*, **64**, 76–79.
2. Berwick DM. (1989) Continuous improvement as an ideal in health care. *New England Journal of Medicine* **320**, 53–55.
3. California Mental Health Planning Council (2005). *Partnerships for Quality: California's Statewide Quality Improvement System.* www.dhcs.ca.gov/services/MH /Documents/Partnership%20for%20Quality.pdf
4. Tondora J, Miller R. (2009) *Person-Centered Care Questionnaire.* Yale Program for Recovery and Community Health, New Haven, CT.
5. Campbell-Orde T, Chamberlin J, Carpenter J *et al.* (eds) (2005). *Measuring the Promise of Recovery: A Compendium of Recovery Measures.* The Evaluation Center at HSRI, Cambridge, MA.
6. O'Connell M, Tondora J, Croog G *et al.* (2005). *Recovery Self-Assessment.* In Campbell-Orde T, Chamberlin J, Carpenter J *et al.* (eds) *Measuring the Promise of Recovery: A Compendium of Recovery Measures.* The Evaluation Center at HSRI, Cambridge, MA.

7. Burgess P, Pirkis J, Coombs T, Rosen A. (2011). Assessing the value of existing recovery measures for routine use in Australian mental health services. *Australian and New Zealand Journal of Psychiatry* **45**, 267–80.

8. Williams J, Leamy M, Bird V *et al.* (2012). Measures of the recovery orientation of mental health services: systematic review. *Social Psychiatry and Psychiatric Epidemiology* **47**, 1827–1835.

9. Jonikas J, Cook J, Fudge N *et al.* (2005). Charting a Meaningful Life: Planning Ownership in Person/Family-Centered Planning. Paper presented at SAMHSA's National Consensus Initiative on Person/Family Center Planning Meeting on December, 8th 2005, Washington, DC.

10. Council on Quality and Leadership. (2005) Council on Quality and Leadership. www.thecouncil.org/assets/0/235/238/7dec14a120f3411b8aab688672dcc858.pdf.

11. Ridgway, P, Press, A. (2004). *Assessing the recovery-orientation of your mental health program: A user's guide for the Recovery-Enhancing Environment Scale (REE).* Version 1. University of Kansas, School of Social Welfare, Office of Mental Health Training and Research, Lawrence, Kansas.

12. Roe, D, Mashiach-Eizenberg, M, Corrigan, P (2012). Confirmatory factor analysis of the brief version of the Recovery Assessment Scale. *Journal of Nervous & Mental Disease,* **200**, 847–851.

13. Rogers, E, Chamberlin, J, Ellison M, *et al.* (1997). A consumer-constructed scale to measure empowerment among users of mental health services. *Psychiatric Services,* **48**, 1042–1047.

14. Herth, K (1992). Abbreviated instrument to measure hope: development and psychometric evaluation. *Journal of Advanced Nursing,* **17**, 1251–1259.

15. Gagne C. (2002). *Characteristics of recovery-oriented mental health programs: Can I recognize one if I see one?* Innovations in Recovery & Rehabilitation: The Decade of the Person Conference. Boston, MA (October 24–26, 2002).

16. Onken SJ, Dumont JM, Ridgway P *et al.* (2002) *Mental Health Recovery: What Helps and What Hinders? A National Research Project for the Development of Recovery Facilitating System Performance Indicators. Phase One Research Report.* National Association of State Mental Health Program Directors National Technical Assistance Center, Alexandria, VA.

17. Jacobson N, Curtis L. (2000) Recovery as policy in mental health services: strategies emerging from the states. *Psychiatric Rehabilitation Journal* **23**, 333–341.

18. Young AS, Forquer SL, Tran A *et al.* (2000). Identifying clinical competencies that support rehabilitation and empowerment in individuals with severe mental illness. *Journal of Behavioral Health Services Research* **27**, 321–333.

19. Chinman M, Young AS, Rowe M *et al.* (2003). An instrument to assess competencies of providers treating severe mental illness. *Mental Health Services Research* **5**, 97–108.

20. Mental Health Commission. (2001) *Recovery Competencies for New Zealand Mental Health Workers.* Mental Health Commission, Wellington, NZ.

21. Selleck V, Knight E, Migas N *et al.* (2005) Consumers at the Center: True Transformation or More Reform without Change? Accessed from: http://mhepinc.org/documents/consumers_at_the_center.html

22. Davidson L, Ridgway P, O'Connell M.J & Kirk T.A.: Transforming mental health care through participation of the recovery community. In Nelson G, Kloos B, & Ornelas J, (Eds.), Community psychology and community mental health: Towards transformative change. New York: Oxford University Press, in press.

Answers to the Learning Assessment:

1. T
2. T
3. F
4. T
5. T

Module 8: PCCP implementation: Common concerns and person-centered responses

Goal

This concluding module attempts to tie up several loose ends that may remain from the previous modules. Though there are many factors *facilitating* the adoption of rigorous person-centered care planning (PCCP), there are also common misperceptions that hinder its implementation. This module is dedicated to a discussion of these frequently identified concerns that mental health practitioners and system leaders often express regarding the introduction of PCCP. In addition, alternative ways of thinking about, and responding to, around each of these areas are presented. Given the heightened sensitivity to safety issues in the current climate, it also focuses in depth on the issue of the perceived risks involved in a shift toward PCCP.

Learning Objectives

After completing this module, you will be better able to:

- identify and address the most common concerns that practitioners have had about adopting PCCP processes in their practice;
- have a realistic sense of the risks entailed in promoting service user autonomy within the context of PCCP and appreciate the need for appropriate risk assessment and management;
- understand the purpose and function of psychiatric advance directives and other self-care tools in minimizing risk in a way that preserves autonomy while promoting safety for all parties.

Partnering for Recovery in Mental Health: A Practical Guide to Person-Centered Planning, First Edition.
Janis Tondora, Rebecca Miller, Mike Slade and Larry Davidson.
© 2014 John Wiley & Sons, Ltd. Published 2014 by John Wiley & Sons, Ltd.

Common Practitioner Concerns

This section addresses 10 of the most common concerns that direct care staff, program managers, and agency administrators have raised in relation to the adoption of person-centered care planning (PCCP) in their organizations [1]. These concerns are summarized in Table 8.1, and range from the practical (*Will we be able to bill for a person-centered plan? How will we ever find the time to do PCCP?*) to the more philosophical (*Is it too "risky" to support people with serious mental illnesses in making their own decisions? How does this fit with my role as a clinical practitioner?*). As mentioned earlier while introducing the broader notion of recovery-oriented practice (of which PCCP is one of several key components) [2], a primary concern identified by these stakeholders is that of potentially increasing risk, and decreasing safety, through the promotion of personal choice. This module spends additional time addressing this issue and offering recovery-oriented alternatives to current, coercive interventions.

Table 8.1   The Top 10 Practitioner/Administrator Concerns about Person-Centered Care Planning

10	Emphasizing client choice inevitably devalues clinical knowledge and professional expertise.
9	While person-centered care planning may be useful, it is really the responsibility of nonclinical practitioners. It has little to do with treatment.
8	We do "recovery" already; our care is already person-centered.
7	The care plan is not really that important and is not actually used to drive care. It is just for accreditation and reimbursement purposes.
6	Person-centered care planning is supposed to be based on people's own goals, but many people with serious mental illnesses give up on any goals. They are doing their best just to get through each day and may not want to make any changes. Who is to say that they have to be working toward "goals"?
5	Don't the principles of person-centered care contradict the current emphasis on using evidence-based practices?
4	Person-centered care makes sense only when the person has accepted treatment and it has been effective. But most people with severe mental illnesses are too disabled to pursue recovery goals. The first step is getting their clinical issues under control. Later, they can make their own choices.
3	Person-centered care planning takes time and is labor intensive. With high caseloads, practitioners simply do not have the time it takes to do it.
2	Person-centered care planning is not consistent with the concept of "medical necessity" and therefore will not be reimbursed. It is also not consistent with the stipulations of regulatory and accrediting bodies.
1	Allowing people with serious mental illnesses to set their own goals and make their own decisions increases risk and exposes practitioners, and their agencies, to increased liability.

Concern 10. Emphasizing service user choice inevitably devalues clinical knowledge and professional expertise.

This concern has been expressed through comments such as: "Why did I go to medical/ nursing/social work/psychology/etc. school for all of these years if I'm just supposed to do whatever the person wants?" and "But he/she is mentally ill, his/her judgment is impaired, how could he/she know what's best or what he/she needs? And if he/she does, what does he/she need me for?"

In response to these concerns, it is useful to point out that PCCP for persons with mental illness does not require practitioners simply to do whatever an individual wants, any more than patient-centered medicine does for persons with any other medical conditions. Practitioners are still obligated by the ethical principles of their professions to act both in accordance with their training, accrued expertise, and clinical judgment *and* in the best interest of the individual. What is different about PCCP (and patient-centered medicine) is that this care is offered within the context of a collaborative relationship in which the person being served is also recognized as bringing his or her own expertise to the table. This form of expertise, referred to as *expertise by experience*, pertains not to the technical knowledge that the practitioner has but rather to the person's intimate knowledge of his or her own everyday life experiences, his or her needs, values, and preferences, and his or her own aspirations for a life worth living.

The people being served, and their loved ones, bring this knowledge and their concerns to the care planning discussions, while practitioners bring their expertise and skill to bear on assessing, evaluating, diagnosing, educating, informing, and advising the person and his or her loved ones and other allies about the various options they have for treatment, rehabilitation, and support. Decisions about these options are made collaboratively based on the relative benefits and risks/costs of each, on the person's (and family's) personal and cultural values and preferences, and with respect to which options will be most effective in enabling the person to pursue the kind of life he or she will find worth living. On the basis of this plan, practitioners deliver whatever treatment or rehabilitative interventions, or provide whatever supports, they are competent to provide following the nature of the person's conditions, on the practitioner's own training and expertise, and with the informed consent of the person and, if needed, his or her guardian or conservator.

In this sense, it is no more appropriate for the person to assume the role of the practitioner than it is for the practitioner to assume the role of the person, usurping that individual's authority to decide for himself or herself what treatments, interventions, or supports he or she finds will be acceptable. Service users and family members cannot simply tell practitioners what to do, but neither can practitioners simply tell service users or family members what to do and expect them to do it. Under most circumstances (we deal with the exceptions under Concern 1), they have the right to make their own informed decisions. Appreciating this fact, practitioners recognize the need to devote time and attention to educating and informing individuals and families about available and appropriate services and supports and their relative benefits and costs, and providing advice and guidance when requested. And rather than abandoning people or families to what practitioners consider their "poor judgment" when they choose not to take such guidance, practitioners become adept at using persuasion and motivational interventions to encourage them to make better choices over time.

Concern 9. While person-centered care planning may be useful, it is really the responsibility of nonclinical practitioners. It has little to do with treatment.

Representative comments voicing this concern include: "I don't have time to discuss life goals or interests, I barely have the time to conduct a thorough psychiatric evaluation. I leave those to the other staff. My role is to focus on the management of symptoms, that is what I was trained to do," and "Consumers can pursue their interests and get help with their personal goals at the clubhouse/rehab center/housing or voc program. What I provide is clinical care, and it is not within my role to deal with those issues."

As these comments suggest, this concern has multiple components. It is true that no one mental health practitioner will have the requisite expertise to attend to every area of a person's life, ranging from prescribing the right medication to helping the person to find a home and choose an occupation. But PCCP does not require a single practitioner to *do* everything on the care plan for persons with serious mental illnesses. It is more common for the plan to involve several different practitioners with different, complementary, areas of expertise. Physicians and advanced practice nurses know how to assess and diagnose conditions and treat illnesses (among other things), whereas social workers and rehabilitation staff may have been trained to assess, map, develop, and assist people in accessing community resources (among other things). Psychologists may have expertise in cognitive-behavioral psychotherapy, peer staff in establishing trust and role modeling self-care, and still others in legal advocacy or physical health, with plenty of room for overlapping areas of interest. An individual's care should not be driven so much by what expertise happens to be available, however—though that is an important consideration—but by what the person needs and can benefit from given their current priorities and most valued recovery goals.

The PCCP plan provides the overarching framework in which those discussions are held and decisions are made about what this person needs and can benefit from at this point in time. Different needs and aspirations may be addressed by different people—including the person himself or herself and his or her natural supporters—but everyone involved in a person's care needs to know what role he or she is to play within the broader context of the person's life and how his or her role will interact with, influence, and be influenced by, the roles of others. I may view my role as primarily that of assessing symptoms and prescribing effective medications, but if I do not know that my client is at the same time trying to go back to school or to get a job, I will be missing out on important information that would influence decisions about dosage, administration schedules, and side effect profiles. Administering a sedating medication at night may work well for someone who is having difficulty sleeping, but may not work well for someone who has to get up on time to make it to an early class. Furthermore, a medication that is framed as useful in the person's efforts to succeed at school (e.g., if we turn down the volume of the voices, you will be able to concentrate better on what the instructor is saying) is much more likely to be taken as prescribed than a medication that poses additional obstacles to what the person is trying to achieve (e.g., the tremors I get from this pill make it hard for me to count out change from the register).

PCCPs help to ensure that we are not wasting our time trying to get people to accept treatments or other interventions they do not want and that all of the interventions and supports we do provide are integrated within the overall context of the person's everyday life. So while a physician may not be the one to help a person find a home, it is important that he or she knows that the person is currently homeless, as this will influence other decisions about the person's care. Similarly, while a job coach will not be the one to prescribe medications, he or she will need to be attentive to both the effects and side effects of the medications being prescribed, as these may impact on the person's ability to get to work on time and to perform the tasks of the job. For a person to benefit from the collective expertise of the different practitioners involved in his or her care, it is important for all of those practitioners to be "on the same page." In this case, the "page" is the PCCP that stipulates the respective roles of each of the practitioners involved, along with action steps for the person and for his or her natural supporters.

Refer back to the example of Mr. Gonzalez presented in Module 1. Mr. Gonzalez is a man living with bipolar disorder who wishes to be the best father he can be to his children, but whose symptoms of mania have led him to behave in a manner that has frightened his children and alienated his wife. A traditional treatment plan might focus exclusively on clinical issues to be addressed by a psychiatrist (e.g., compliance with medications and reduction of mania) with little, or no, mention of the man's ultimate goal of reunification with his family, which might be viewed as a task for a social worker (and listed separately on a social work plan). We suggest that this lack of connection between treatment and personally valued life goals is one reason why attrition and dropout rates are so high in outpatient mental health care [3–5]. For practitioners to offer more responsive and individualized care, the care planning process needs to be driven by the person's life goals rather than by the practitioner's specific training or professional discipline. In person-centered care, we no longer have a clinical goal that exists independent of a meaningful outcome in a person's life. The goal on the care plan—whether one is a psychiatrist or a social worker—is the same; for example, Mr. Gonzalez wants to reconnect with his family and be a good father. Each practitioner then assists Mr. Gonzalez based on his or her respective role and skills, with the social worker offering family counseling and the psychiatrist prescribing medications that can stabilize his mood and educating Mr. Gonzalez about ways to monitor his own early warning signs to prevent future episodes of behavioral dyscontrol. While such a difference may seem trivial to the psychiatrist, it may make all the difference in Mr. Gonzalez's motivations for taking the medication that is prescribed (e.g., to reconnect with his family and be a good father as opposed to treating his bipolar disorder).

In summary, assertions by clinical practitioners that "those things (i.e., the pursuit of meaningful jobs, relationships, leisure interests) are important but they are really the focus of the clubhouse or the peer services team" serve to perpetuate a fragmented model of care where the obligation to deliver recovery-promoting services is deemed to be the sole responsibility of a specialized program or distinct group of individuals. While certain programs (e.g., peer-operated or rehabilitation programs) may be uniquely positioned to be leaders in recovery-oriented change efforts, these ideas must reshape how business is done in

ALL parts of a system in order for meaningful transformation to occur. Recovery-oriented, person-centered care is not an "add-on" to be passed off to any one discipline or program. Rather, it implies profound changes across all staff roles, from clinicians through administrative assistants and psychiatrists to the CFO!

Concern 8. We do "recovery" already; our care is already person-centered.

Some practitioners take offense at the notion that the care they offer is not already recovery-oriented and person-centered. They object to the insinuation that they do not "take the person into account," are not respectful of their service users, or do not tailor their interventions to each individual. If there are limitations placed on the degree to which their practice can be so, it is not their "fault," but is rather due to the seemingly arbitrary and artificial constraints placed on them by the agencies and systems in which they work. There is simply not enough time to get to know the person: the paperwork requirements supersede their desire to be genuinely helpful, and/or the funders of services limit what practitioners can do and for how long.

We agree that caring and compassionate practitioners do already make concerted efforts to "take the person into account" and that many organizational and systemic barriers to person-centered care exist that will need to be changed dramatically in order to improve the quality of care practitioners can provide. These recognitions do not lead necessarily to resignation or to the conclusion that practice cannot be made more person-centered within current constraints, however. You most likely would not be reading this manual if you thought no steps could be taken to make your practice both more person-centered and more effective and gratifying. So *in addition* to listening empathically to the person and tailoring the care one provides to each individual, we suggest that PCCP involves the use of new tools and strategies that practitioners may have some familiarity with, but which generally are not employed routinely in practice. These include comprehensive and structured interests and strengths assessments; the inclusion of the person's natural supporters and legal advocates in the care planning process; articulation of clearly defined short- and long-term personal goals with measurable objectives; assignment of responsibility for different tasks and action steps to different members of the care team, including the person in recovery; prioritization of natural, integrated settings over those designed solely for persons labeled with serious mental illnesses; and the use of tools such as psychiatric advanced directives, shared decision-making aids, and supported employment, housing, education, socialization, and parenting.

Thus, while many practitioners strive to attend to each person as a unique individual, there are many strategies and tools (some new, some longstanding) that are underutilized and whose consistent use in routine practice could significantly advance the implementation of a more person-centered model of care planning. Several concrete and specific indicators of PCCP are spelled out in detail in the Person-Centered Care Questionnaire (PCCQ) included at the end of Module 7. Practitioners are encouraged to complete the PCCQ in order to assess the degree to which their current practice already adheres to the principles outlined in this manual and to identify those areas in which they might take new risks to enhance their services.

Concern 7. The care plan is not really that important and is not actually used to drive care. It is just for accreditation and reimbursement purposes.

Practitioners may object to such attention being paid, and such importance being given, to what they view as largely a bureaucratic requirement, saying things such as: "Why are you focusing on a piece of paper that has little to nothing to do with the care I provide to my clients? It is for the chart, not for the person. Does it really matter?"

In practice, treatment plans have often been and are technical documents that have to be completed to satisfy accrediting (what is referred to in some settings as *commissioning*) or reimbursement bodies and typically have not been and are not useful either to the practitioner or to the person using the services. In such cases, the plan is completed and filed in the medical record and plays little, if any, role in actually guiding care. We do not believe that anyone would argue that this is an ideal way of providing services or occupying the time and talents of dedicated practitioners. While we recognize this is still the unfortunate reality of most treatment plans written in today's systems of care, we propose that the truly person-centered plan—one created through a process of partnership, shared discovery, and thoughtful action planning—has the potential to be a powerful transformative tool. Rather than being a bureaucratic document that takes time away from the real work of direct care, the co-creation of the PCCP is best thought of as a central intervention in and of itself, as it becomes the very heart of the work and the therapeutic and healing process.

PCCP emphasizes the need for the individual to enter into a collaborative process with practitioners and natural supports to explore and identify the goals and objectives that will promote the person's recovery and improve his or her quality of life. The resulting care plan is a roadmap for pursuing valued life goals and the milestones that are achieved along the way (i.e., short-term objectives) serve to give both the individual and his or her practitioners and loved ones the critical experiences of success and forward momentum needed to overcome the inevitable frustrations and setbacks that are encountered along the road ahead. In this sense, the plan becomes a useful tool that has direct relevance in guiding the work of the person and his or her team over time. It can be consulted as needed in order to ensure that all parties stay on course and revised as often as needed if the person reaches certain landmarks or has to bypass or work around roadblocks met along the way or if the person chooses to select a new destination.

Concern 6. Person-centered care planning is supposed to be based on people's own goals, but many people with serious mental illnesses give up on any goals. They are doing their best just to get through each day and may not want to make any changes. Who is to say that they have to be working toward "goals?"

Change is admittedly hard for everyone, and caring practitioners who work with individuals who are seriously disabled by mental illnesses and the discrimination that has resulted from it are right to ask: "But what if my clients don't have goals?" or to remark that: "When I ask my clients what their goals are they just give me a blank stare. They seem comfortable where they are, who am I to tell them that they have to change?"

Here it is important to acknowledge that most people do not live their lives explicitly in terms of "goals." We are using this concept as a term of art to convey important ideas to practitioners, but are reluctant to use this term explicitly with persons in recovery or their loved ones, especially without being clear about what we mean. We all have dreams and aspirations, we all find enjoyment, pleasure, and meaning in some activities and pursuits more than others, but seldom do most of us take the time to break these down into the various steps that will be required for us to engage in them. Similarly, while many people with serious mental illnesses will not have explicit goals and may well not know how to answer questions that ask them about goals, they nonetheless will have some ideas about *what could make their lives better*. But before they share these ideas with anyone, they will have to feel some sense of trust and confidence that this information will be used in their best interest, to help them, rather than for other, less benevolent purposes.

For many persons who have been receiving psychiatric care for a while, for instance, the seemingly simple question of "What do you think would make your life better?" might strike them as odd and unexpected. They might even give voice to this reaction by saying: "Why would you care about my life all of a sudden? I thought you only cared about my symptoms." Rather than viewing this as a sign of being paranoid, or as a response that reflects the person's lack of goals, we should consider the context in which this question is being asked. Other barriers to goal identification might be the negative symptoms associated with schizophrenia and/or the demoralization that accompanies living with a serious mental illness and being subjected to the societal stigma and discrimination associated with it. In the wake of such devastation, it is understandable how it might be difficult for some people to identify and share their personal aspirations and interests, and why they might be reluctant to dare to hope for a better life. In such cases, it may require patience and persistence on the part of both practitioners and the person's loved ones in encouraging him or her to imagine what might make his or her life better than it currently is. With so many of his or her previous dreams having been interrupted by illness and/or dashed by the legacy of the low expectations we have had for persons with serious mental illnesses, it may at first feel dangerous or scary to allow themselves to dream once again.

When facing such circumstances, practitioners need to conceptualize one of their first steps as assisting the person to get back in touch with his or her previous interests and talents and to draw on these to imagine a brighter tomorrow. What interested them when they were younger, what activities did they use to enjoy, what gave them a sense of pride or mastery? Had they been too distant from, or uninterested in looking back at, life before the illness, how would they like to be spending their time now on a day-to-day basis? Do they, for example, want to work and make money? Or, would they perhaps like to have a better place to live, or one closer to activities they might enjoy participating in? What gives them pleasure or a sense of success? This type of dialogue differs significantly from the more restrictive conversation in which the person has been expected merely to report on symptoms and side effects or patterns of eating, sleeping, and taking medications. Using strength-based inquiry to inspire hope and to support people in goal setting is a process that requires both clinical skill and perhaps a willingness to step outside the comfort zone of our inherited professional discourse.

Concern 5. Don't the principles of person-centered care contradict the current emphasis on using evidence-based practices?

Given that advances in PCCP are relatively recent and may be new to many practitioners, it is fairly common for some practitioners to wonder about the "evidence base" supporting this practice. They may even see contradictions between recovery-oriented and evidence-based practices, struggling to know what to do. They often ask, for example, "Am I supposed to follow clinical guidelines and offer evidence-based practices or am I supposed to do what the client says he or she wants? What if those two things are not the same? I can't do both."

As noted already in Concern 10, PCCP does not equate to "giving the client whatever he or she wants." Practitioners practice within their areas of expertise, offering interventions for which they have been trained and in which they are skilled. What PCCP requires is for the delivery (or not) of these services to be based on a collaborative decision-making process in which the person plays a central role in weighing the evidence and determining which services and supports will likely be most useful in helping him or her to have the kind of life he or she will find worth living. Rather than being in conflict with "evidence-based practices," this emphasis on the central role of the person's own needs, values, and preferences in decision making is actually one of the three core components of evidence-based medicine, from which the emphasis on evidence-based practices has arisen. Evidence-based medicine refers to practitioners using (i) their own clinical judgment in combination with (ii) educating patients about the accumulated evidence in support of the various options available to treat their condition, while (iii) respecting each patient's right to make his or her own health care decisions (except in extenuating circumstances). This definition is also consistent with the definition of "patient-centered medicine" offered by the US Institute of Medicine (IOM) [6], which, over a decade ago, established "care that is respectful of and responsive to individual patient preferences, needs, and values, and ensures that patient values guide all clinical decisions" as the expected standard.

Concern 4. Person-centered care makes sense only when the person has accepted treatment and it has been effective. But many people with severe mental illnesses are too disabled to pursue recovery goals. The first step is getting their clinical issues under control. Later, they can make their own choices.

Practitioners who work with persons with serious mental illnesses may initially consider PCCP to be a luxury that can not be afforded until well along in a person's recovery, once the person is "clinically stable" or relatively asymptomatic. They might suggest that: "Person-centered care sounds great for people who are well on their way to recovery, but the people I see are so ill, they're not ready to be in the 'driver's seat' of their own care. First they need to accept having a mental illness, accept their need for treatment, take their medications. Then, once they've got the illness under some control, we can revisit goals like getting to school, a job, or a new place to live."

Undoubtedly, there are times when persons with serious mental illnesses want to be taken care of by others, just as there are times when people who do not have serious mental illnesses want to be taken care of. In the case of serious mental illnesses, such times may be when they are experiencing acute episodes and/or are in extreme distress. On the basis of first-person accounts of people in recovery and on the collective wisdom of various laws and accrediting or commissioning bodies, we are not to take this preference for being taken care of for short periods to generalize to the remainder of the person's life. The majority of persons with serious mental illnesses will spend only about 5% of their adult lives in acute episodes and/or extreme distress, and the remaining 95% will be spent in periods of relative symptomatic and functional stability [7]. It is during this 95% of the time that PCCP is best carried out, including planning, through the use of proactive crisis plans or psychiatric advance directives (PADs) (discussed in greater detail later in this module), for how the person would like to be cared for and supported during that 5% of the time when he or she may be too incapacitated to make his or her own decisions.

For those people for whom the 95% rule does not appear to apply and/or who may seem too disabled to make their own decisions on an ongoing basis, we suggest that there remains a significant amount of latitude for practitioners to elicit and be guided by the person's own values, needs, and preferences. It is equally important for persons with significant disabilities to have as much choice as possible as it is for anyone else, even if that choice has to be based on a restricted range of options due to the person's condition and circumstances. Simple examples of how this principle can be honored in practice are in asking people in institutional settings how they would like to spend their time, what and with whom they would like to eat, and what activities would give them some degree of pleasure, rather than insisting they first participate in treatment and other activities that have proven not to be effective for them in the past. Even if these core treatment activities did have some effectiveness, to expect someone to solely and rigidly move through a predetermined continuum of care is, we suggest, a subtle yet pernicious form of coercion that undermines the sense of agency needed for recovery.

Unfortunately, despite the positive changes brought about over the past decade or so by system transformation, it is still not uncommon for individuals to be expected to jump through clinical "hoops" and demonstrate clinical stability before moving on to pursue broader life goals (e.g., requiring 6 months of medication compliance as a prerequisite for referral to supported employment or dictating a certain level of compliance with unit groups before being allowed to participate in a hospital's treatment mall rehabilitation program). Ironically, engagement in these personally preferred activities is often the factor that ultimately increases the person's desires to acknowledge and begin to work on many of the "core" clinical issues that may interfere with their progress. If treatment is not viewed as moving the person closer to the things he or she values in life, if it does not increase the person's sense of meaning, purpose, or pleasure in life, then what motivation does the person have to "accept" having an illness or needing treatment?

Finally, the consumer/survivor/service user literature has argued that much of what practitioners view as apathy, passivity, or a lack of motivation in persons with serious mental illnesses is actually due to "learned helplessness" [8] stemming from years of having other people take over control and decision-making authority for their lives. Just as the process of sharing power and responsibility in care planning may at times pose a disconcerting shift in roles among some mental health practitioners, many persons with serious mental illnesses may truly want to exert greater control over their lives but feel unprepared to do so. To the degree that this is a contributor to a person not wanting to make his or her own decisions or to take a backseat in care planning, the process of reinstilling a sense of control, competence, and confidence in a person's own decision-making capacity will require time, incremental successes, and provision of mentoring and skill-building opportunities specific to the process of PCCP.

Concern 3. Person-centered care planning takes time and is labor intensive. With high caseloads, practitioners simply do not have the time it takes to do it.

Harried and overworked practitioners understandably complain: "I have to fill out piles of paperwork on loads of clients on a tight timeline and there's just no way I can discuss everything with each client first—especially when the client doesn't show up half the time! How can I get my paperwork in, keep my supervisor off my back, and still do PCCP?"

We acknowledge that mental health practice in today's fiscal climate balances on razor-thin margins. Budget deficits, or shifting political priorities, have led to stretching limited resources, making this seem like an unpropitious time to advocate for the expansion of PCCP, which might seem at first to make additional demands on the limited time practitioners have. Yet research shows that while having intensive conversations regarding the life context, aspirations, goals, and strengths of individuals may require more time up front, this investment in developing a collaborative relationship tends to be time and labor saving in the long run [9]. Not only are people more likely to attend appointments that seem relevant to what they want out of life—thus cutting down on the high rate of "no shows" in outpatient clinics [10]—but practitioners are also more likely to elicit the much needed information that saves them from wasting time on activities that may not benefit the individual (e.g., encouraging compliance with medications that are not effective) and enables them to focus their efforts where they are most likely to have an impact. In addition, shifting the focus to the person's own responsibility for and role in recovery allows practitioners to shift from an onerous "do to" or "do for" perspective to a collaborative "do with" perspective, fostering increasing independence on the part of the individual and shifting care from a reliance on shrinking institutional resources and solutions toward more of an integration of natural community connections and supports, which in turn lead to increasing integration of the person into the life of his or her community.

Finally, program evaluation findings on PCCP models suggest that this approach to care can interrupt costly cycles of reactive crisis response, leading to reductions in hospitalizations, incarcerations, and assaultive or self-injurious behavior [11]. We suggest that the frequent management of such crisis situations stretches systems and practitioners far more than the additional time needed to engage in more proactive and collaborative PCCP. Ultimately, PCCPs may take more time to create than the cookie-cutter documents that still populate many medical records in mental health systems across the globe. However, we view this as time well spent and suggest that it is a prudent investment in improving the quality of our partnerships with, and the quality of life among, persons in recovery.

Concern 2. Person-centered care planning is not consistent with the concept of "medical necessity" and therefore will not be reimbursed. It is also not consistent with the stipulations of regulatory and accrediting or commissioning bodies.

Worried practitioners have expressed the fear that implementation of PCCP will have dire consequences for their agencies, and therefore for their livelihoods. They have argued:

"We can't lose our accreditation and our income. Our funders and regulators will not allow us to focus on 'recovery' goals. They're primarily interested in our treating illnesses. We'll be cited or have paybacks."

Our response to this concern builds on the response we gave to Concern 9, related to how PCCP seems to challenge, if not violate, professional roles and identities. In this case, the concern is that PCCP is not consistent with the traditional, so-called narrow "medical model" and the regulatory and funding bodies that have historically governed mental health care. Our response to this concern is complex, as the issues involved are themselves complex.

First, regulatory, accrediting, and governmental bodies have been for some time, and are currently, ahead of everyday practice regarding the importance placed on person-centered and goal-directed care. Individually tailored care oriented to each person's unique condition and circumstances and focused on the achievement of each person's expressed goals has been their mandate for years, even prior to the advent of person-centered care in mental health *per se*. In addition, care is to be delivered only with the informed consent of the person (in all but the most extenuating of circumstances) and is expected to be strength-based, culturally competent, and responsive to each person's individual life context, and all of these domains are to be documented adequately in the person's medical record. Indeed, much of the funding for the work on which this manual is based was awarded by the US Centers for Medicare and Medicaid Services (CMS), the bastion of health care that is responsible for the very notion of "medical necessity."

These facts do not negate practitioners' concerns, however, that PCCP principles do not seem to translate readily into the categories and concepts of conventional care plans. Were they to do so, though, we would have to question how much their introduction can effect actual and substantial changes in the way we provide care. Efforts must therefore be made to reconceptualize care plans and documentation tools to become person-centered, strength-based, and goal-directed. Doing so does not minimize the importance of illness, deficits, and problems, but does reframe them within the context of the person's overall life. That said, it remains true that CMS, for instance, will not (yet) provide reimbursement for certain services or supports that some persons with serious mental illnesses desire and will find useful. For the time being—until, that is, these regulatory, accrediting, and funding bodies move further in the direction of self-directed care and flexible funding—other sources of funding will need to be identified for these kinds of services (e.g., transportation or job coaching) or they will need to be secured beyond the parameters of the formal mental health system in the community at large. Ultimately, this may be a solution that will be both cost-effective and consistent with the desire of persons in recovery, who seldom wish to live out the entirety of their lives within the mental health system.

Even presently, though, it is common for practitioners to view regulatory and funding bodies as more formidable barriers to providing person-centered care than they in fact need to be. We believe this derives from two fundamental misconceptions. First is the belief that person-centered planning is somehow "soft." Second is the belief that funders will not pay for life goals such as helping someone to finish school or return to work.

Contrary to the common myth that person-centered planning is "soft," emerging practice guidelines explicitly call for the documentation of (i) comprehensive clinical formulations that include (ii) mental health-related barriers that interfere with functioning along with (iii) strengths and resources that can be used to achieve (iv) short-term and measurable objectives using (v) clearly articulated interventions that spell out who is doing what on what timeline and for what purpose [12]. On the basis of hundreds of chart reviews done by the authors and our colleagues, we suggest that these standards for PCCP documentation are on par with, if not superior to, the level of rigor that currently exists in most care plans.

Second, the belief that funders will not pay for nonclinical goals is actually a correct one; not, however, because of the nature of the goal itself, but because of the fact that funders do not pay for *goals* at all. Rather, they pay mental health practitioners for the interventions and professional services and supports they provide. In our experience, these services and supports will be funded if they help people overcome documented mental health and/or addiction-related barriers that interfere with their everyday functioning and the attainment of their valued life (i.e., "recovery") goals. In other words, interventions may be considered "medically necessary" when they are required following the impact of a mental illness on one or more functional domains in a person's everyday life. Social isolation offers an excellent example. In most cases, it is understood to be both a sequela of mental illness that causes suffering and a factor that impairs overall health. On this basis, interventions that aim to increase a person's social functioning can most often be reimbursed should they be required by the nature of the person's illness and consistent with the person's own desires to have a broader social network, including the goal of "I want to find a partner and get married."

This is admittedly a broad-brush review and we acknowledge that each locality may be subject to its own unique funding and regulatory expectations, a full discussion of which is beyond the scope of this manual. However, we maintain that medical necessity and PCCP are not incompatible constructs and that care plans can be created in partnership with persons in recovery and their loved ones while still maintaining rigorous standards in treatment and care planning and documentation.

Concern 1. Allowing people with serious mental illnesses to set their own goals and make their own decisions increases risk and exposes practitioners, and their agencies, to increased liability.

Fully aware of their agency's and supervisor's concerns with risk management and liability exposure, practitioners may well wonder: "Isn't impaired judgment one of the core characteristics of serious mental illness? If I give my clients choices, and they make bad ones, won't I be the one held responsible? When things go wrong, I'll get the blame."

PCCP does not override a practitioner's ethical and societal obligation to intervene on a person's or the community's behalf should someone pose a serious and imminent threat to self or others. In such cases, just as in the case of an automobile accident or traumatic brain injury, health care practitioners are sanctioned to intervene on the person's behalf without getting prior consent. In psychiatry, as in most other branches of medicine, however, such cases are the extremes and the exceptions, not the norm. Consistent with our response to Concern 4 above, research suggests that most people with most mental illnesses pose few if any risks most of the time. Risk can be exacerbated by substance use and by nonadherence to medication, but even then the risk posed by people with serious mental illnesses pales in comparison to the risks they face from others, as it is much more common for a person with a serious mental illness to be the victim of a crime than to be a perpetrator [13, 14].

What these data suggest is that heightened concerns about increased risk and liability are misplaced when applied to most persons with serious mental illnesses most of the time. In the circumstances in which they are warranted, prudent risk assessment and management are central and crucial aspects of effective care. PCCP does not do away with, or replace, this need. What PCCP insists, though, is that when risks are determined *not* to be present, as is the case the vast majority of the time, that the person be encouraged to make his or her own choices, as he or she is entitled to by law. Otherwise, coercion in the absence of risk places undue restrictions on the liberty of persons with serious mental illnesses, with individual liberty being one of the most important and central values held in democratic societies.

But how do we respond to the objection that persons with serious mental illnesses will make bad choices or demonstrate poor judgment when left up to their own devices, more as a result of their illness than as a genuine exercise of their autonomy? Family members or guardians, in particular, may insist that their loved one should not be allowed to make certain decisions that they know this person would not make were he or she well, that is, not under the sway of a mental illness. While it is certainly understandable for family members or guardians to have such firm convictions—and they are fully in their rights to try to persuade their loved one to make different choices—practitioners are obligated ethically first and foremost (in the absence of imminent risk) to honor the decisions of the service user.

Fortunately, and despite the stereotype about impaired judgment, research has shown that people with serious mental illnesses on the whole make decisions about their care in ways very similar to people with other medical conditions. That is, some people with mental illnesses make good decisions most of the time, some make good decisions some of the time, and some make good decisions only occasionally. But this is also true of the general population [15]. People who do not have a mental illness are in general no better at decision making than people who do, meaning that people who have a mental illness are in general no worse at decision making than people who do not. Currently, the only legal or statutory basis for interfering with an individual's personal sovereignty (other than in situations of serious risk) is when the person has been determined by a judge to be incapable of making his or her own decisions and, as a result, has been assigned a legal guardian or conservator of person. Even in those cases, the law often insists that the judge outline those specific areas in which the guardian or conservator is authorized to override the person's own choices. Short of this, the majority of individuals with serious mental illnesses retain both the right and the responsibility of making their own decisions and of dealing with, and learning from, the outcomes of those decisions. As Patricia Deegan has reminded us in arguing for people to retain "the dignity of risk and the right to fail" [16], that is the way most adults learn most things in life.

Where, then, does this leave the compassionate practitioner who wishes to support a person in making his or her own choices, but who fears that the person is making detrimental decisions that are likely to jeopardize his or her recovery and well-being? There can be many such dilemmas in practice, including people who choose not to take medications that appeared to be helping them, people who remain in relationships with others who physically and/or emotionally abuse them, people who keep making the same bad decisions over and over again and appear not to be learning from their mistakes, and so on. In these and similar situations, we argue strenuously *against* the stance that practitioners should abandon service users to their bad choices or sit silently by on the sidelines in the name of being "person-centered" or in the hope that the person will eventually learn from suffering the "natural consequences" of a pattern of apparently self-defeating choices. Honoring the "dignity of risk and the right to fail" does not equal neglect. Rather, in keeping with the emerging best practices in recovery-oriented care [20], we suggest that the role of the practitioner in such situations is to remain fully engaged with the person in exploring what a given choice means to him or her, why it seems so important, and what the potential pros and cons are, and in brainstorming alternative choices, ensuring that the person has all the information necessary to make a fully informed decision. Practitioners are also encouraged to use motivational interventions to identify, explore, and resolve ambivalence the person may feel about his or her decisions, hoping that gradually, over time, he or she will make those choices that are in his or her best interest.

Barring any immediate safety concerns, though, it is the person's decision to make, just as it is in other health care arenas. Following the kind of collaborative explorations and discussions described above, the person may, in fact, arrive at different decisions from where he or she began. On the other hand, practitioners may gain additional insights into why it is important for the person to make the decisions he or she makes, and might well be surprised when those decisions turn out to be less detrimental than he or she originally thought. In addition, compromises become possible within the context of trusting relationships when the person fully believes that the practitioner wants what is best for him or her (as opposed to what is expedient or safe). However, we recognize that there also will be circumstances in which the person and the practitioner will need to "agree to disagree" for the time being, while remaining nonetheless engaged in a caring relationship. At these times, practitioners may remain concerned that they are failing to meet their ethical obligations or exposing themselves to liability by not insisting that the individual do what the practitioner deems best or even by stopping the individual from doing what he or she wants to do. The most prudent actions in these cases, when there is no evidence of serious and imminent risk, is for the practitioner to document fully and faithfully in the person's medical record the discussions that he or she has had with the person, including his or her own efforts to communicate concern, to provide necessary information and support to persuade the individual to act differently, to propose alternative courses of action, and, of course, to assess risk.

While every situation needs to be evaluated on a case-by-case basis, and every person is different and will pose unique challenges and dilemmas, we believe that this represents a balanced perspective that respects both the person's right to make his or her own decisions and the practitioner's need to ensure that he or she has done his or her due diligence and upheld his or her professional and ethical obligations.

Within the context of a recovery-oriented, risk-management approach, there are tools that practitioners can use to be proactive in anticipating crises and in supporting individuals to plan ahead for those circumstances in which they may temporarily lose the capacity to make their own decisions. For example, an innovative, yet frequently underutilized tool, is the PAD, legal documents supported by the 1991 Patient Self-Determination Act, PADs allow a person to indicate his or her preferences for mental health and physical health treatment in the event that he or she is unable to communicate these preferences

> *I* pretty much carry my PAD around everywhere. Once … it was really crowded in the ER so I showed intake my psychiatric advance directive and told them that I needed to go somewhere quiet … so that I could calm down … The intake nurse sat with me in a quiet room until I calmed down.
>
> —Person in Recovery on her experience with Psychiatric Advance Directives [17]

at some point in the future. Advance directives, although normally thought of in terms of *physical* healthcare and end-of-life decisions (e.g., living wills), are actually applicable for any period in which a person is deemed incompetent to make treatment decisions—this includes mental health treatment decisions. While the laws governing advance directive differ from state to state (see http://www.nrc-pad.org/ for details), PADs can include both written health care directives as well as the appointment of an authorized proxy (or healthcare decision maker).

Within an advance directive, a person can indicate preferences around a wide range of treatment options including preferences about medications, electroconvulsive therapy (ECT), restraint and seclusion techniques (which can be particularly crucial for individuals with a trauma history), alternatives to hospitalization, persons to contact for information and support, personalized deescalation strategies, arrangements for pet or minor child care, and so on. As illustrated by the below quote, as told to one of the authors during a PCCP training several years ago, the presence (or absence) of an advance directive can have a dramatic impact on a person's experience of care:

> *I will never forget. It was early September and I found my way to my local ER. My symptoms were so intense, I couldn't think straight and could barely speak or string my words together. Even in the middle of that experience, I knew my baby was at her first day of kindergarten and I was not going to be there at the bus to pick her up and it's real rough on my street. I kept trying to tell the nurse, but it wouldn't come out. I finally just lost it ... ended up in restraints in the hallway- all because I didn't have a way to tell them my baby needed me. A few months ago, the Peer Specialist at my clinic helped me fill out an advance directive. It says exactly who needs to be called to take care of my daughter if I ever end up back in the hospital. I hope I never will ... but knowing she will have someone there for her in case, makes all the difference to me.*

PADs and similar self-directed planning tools (e.g., the advance crisis component of Wellness Recovery Action Plan, WRAP, discussed in Module 3) represent innovative ways in which practitioners can step in as needed and take temporary control during a crisis but still do so in a way that allows the individual to maintain as much control and autonomy as possible during a time when it is necessary to temporarily restrict such rights to ensure the person's safety and well-being. In this sense, we consider the routine use of PAD to be an essential practice in PCCP, and strongly encourage their use as innovative, recovery-oriented complements to standard risk-management procedures.

Conclusion

There is one general principle at the heart of person-centered care from which all the content in this manual can be derived. This principle is itself derived from the fundamental assumption that people with mental illnesses have been, are, and will remain people first and foremost, just like everyone else [18]. If people with mental illnesses are first and foremost people, then it follows that person-centered care for people with mental illnesses should first and foremost be similar to, if not exactly the same as, person-centered care for other people, that is, person-centered planning is, at its core, about the attainment of goals that are universal to typical human experiences—goals that appreciate our common humanity, our common aspirations and dreams, and our common sense of responsibility to become contributing members of society [19].

The practice of PCCP as outlined in this manual suggests that the plan of care has the potential to be, and should be, far more than a paperwork requirement. The co-created recovery plan is the manifestation of a respectful partnership as well as a roadmap that outlines a more hopeful vision for the future and how all stakeholders will work together to achieve it. Finally, while the implementation of PCCP inevitably involves encountering and overcoming a range of both practical and philosophical barriers, we hope we have left you with a sense of optimism, that PCCP is, in fact, possible, provided we all recognize our obligation to, in the words of Dale DiLeo [20], "stop accepting what is … and start creating what should be."

Exercises

Exercise 1. Assessing and working around implementation barriers.

Here is a simple data collection tool that summarizes many of the most common PCCP implementation barriers presented throughout this module. Work with a group of your colleagues to distribute the tool to a sample of practitioners in your agency and have them complete the forms anonymously. Collect the completed forms and tally the total number of people identifying each of the PCCP implementation concerns. Consider the following questions:

- What were the three higest and three lowest identified PCCP implementation concerns?
- Were there any surprises when you looked at the quantitative data or qualitative comments?
- What types of interventions might be needed to respond to expressed concerns? Consider:
  - Culture-based interventions that address system-wide attitudes/beliefs/assumptions regarding recovery and person-centered care.
  - Competency-based interventions that target staff competency development in the process and documentation of person-centered plans.
  - Workflow/business-based interventions that address policies and procedures that may need to be clarified and/or modifed to support PCCP.

Person-Centered Care Planning Implementation Concerns

Complete the thought:

The things that I have heard about PCP that concern me (or my agency/system/ supervisees) the most are ... The biggest challenges in implementation are ...

_____

_____

_____

_____

_____

_____

Please check THREE items that represent the biggest implementation challenges in your system:

Common Beliefs/Concerns that Hinder PCP Implementation			
Concern/Challenge	X	Concern/Challenge	X
We would not get paid; regulations prohibit this; we can't write PCPs that meet medical necessity criteria.		PCP devalues clinical expertise; What is the role of the professional if the person is driving the process?	
If given increased choice, consumers may make BAD ones; PCP will expose us to risk/liability issues.		This is important but it is not part of standard clinical care/therapy/treatment; It's what happens at the Clubhouse/Peer Center, and so on.	
Our planning forms do not have the right fields—they are problem driven.		There is not enough time to do PCP; caseloads are too high to work this way.	
Consumers aren't motivated; I can not get them to participate in PCP; they can not identify goals in this way.		Clients are too sick/impaired to partner with us in the planning process.	
PCP does not fit with the focus on rigorous evidence-based practice.		PCP is no different/don't we do it already?	

Learning Assessment

Module 8: PCCP Implementation: Common Concerns and Person-Centered Responses		
Statement	True	False
1. PCCP views both professional knowledge and lived experience as critical in creating a quality person-centered plan.		
2. The person-centered plan is a special plan that gets completed by the rehab department or the peers. It is separate from my master clinical treatment plan.		
3. When practitioners have concerns regarding a change or decision an individual is making, it is best to withhold all comments because the natural consequences will teach him or her a lesson.		
4. Emerging research findings show that person-centered planning can both increase service user engagement and decrease hospital recidivism.		
5. The optimal time to complete a Psychiatric Advance Directive is on admission to a psychiatric emergency department.		
See the Answer Key at the end of the chapter for the correct answers. **Number Correct**		
0 to 2: Don't be discouraged. Learning is an ongoing process! You can review the module for greater knowledge. 3 to 4: Great start. You can continue to use this guide to learn more about planning for recovery. 5: Nice! Use this guide to share what you've learned with others!		

References

1. Tondora J, Miller R, Davidson L. (2012). The top ten concerns about person-centered care planning in mental health systems. *International Journal of Person Centered Medicine* **2**, 410–420.
2. Davidson L, O'Connell MJ, Tondora J et al. (2006). The top ten concerns about recovery encountered in mental health system transformation. *Psychiatric Services* **57**, 640–645.
3. Davidson L, Stayner DA, Lambert S et al. (1997). Phenomenological and participatory research on schizophrenia: recovering the person in theory and practice. *Journal of Social Issues* **53**, 767–784.
4. Kessler RC, Berglund PA, Bruce ML et al. (2001). The prevalence and correlates of untreated serious mental illness. *Health Services Research* **36**, 987–1007.
5. Olfson M, Mojtabai R, Sampson NA et al. (2009). Dropout from outpatient mental health care in the United States. *Psychiatric Services* **60**, 898–907.

6. Institute of Medicine. (2001). *Crossing the quality chasm: A new health system for the 21st century.* National Academy Press, Washington, DC.

7. Wexler B, Davidson L, Styron T, Strauss JS. (2010). Severe and persistent mental illness. In Jacobs S, Griffith EEH. (eds) *40 years of academic public psychiatry.* John Wiley & Sons, Ltd, Chichester, UK, pp. 1–20.

8. Deegan PE. (1992). The independent living movement and people with psychiatric disabilities: Taking back control over our own lives. *Psychosocial Rehabilitation Journal* **15**, 3–19.

9. Wilson A, Childs S. (2002). The relationship between consultation length, process and outcomes in general practice: a systematic review. *British Journal of General Practice* **52**, 1012–1020.

10. Stanhope, V, Ingoglia, C, Schmelter, B. et al. (2013). Impact of person-centered planning and collaborative documentation on treatment adherence. *Psychiatric Services*, **64**, 76–79.

11. Western New York Care Coordination Program Evaluation Results. Retrieved February 12, 2010 from http://www.carecoordination.org/documents/Results%20Book%202010.pdf

12. Adams N, Grieder D. (2004). *Treatment planning for person-centered care: The road to mental health and addiction recovery.* Elsevier Science Publishing, Burlington, Massachusetts.

13. Teplin LA, McClelland GM, Abram KM & Weiner DA. (2005). Crime victimization in adults with severe mental illness: comparison with the National Crime Victimization Survey. *Archives of General Psychiatry* **62**, 911–921.

14. Steadman HJ, Mulvey EP, Monahan J et al. (1998). Violence by people discharged from acute psychiatric impatient facilities and by others in the same neighborhoods. *Archives of General Psychiatry* **55**, 393–401.

15. Bunn MH, O'Connor AM, Tansey MS et al. (1997). Characteristics of clients with schizophrenia who express certainty or uncertainty about continuing treatment with depot neuroleptic medication. *Archives of Psychiatric Nursing* **11**, 238–248.

16. Deegan PE. (1996). Recovery as a journey of the heart. *Psychiatric Rehabilitation Journal* **11**, 11–19.

17. National Resource Center on Psychiatric Advance Directives. Retrieved October 20, 2013 from http://www.nrc-pad.org/pad-stories.

18. Drake R, Deegan PE, Rapp C. (2010). The promise of shared decision making in mental health. *Psychiatric Rehabilitation Journal* **34**, 7–13.

19. Nerney, T. (2004). Quality issues in consumer/family direction. Paper prepared for the SAMHSA Consumer Direction Summit, March 2004.

20. DiLeo, D. (2008). Proceedings of the 14th annual Conference for People with Disabilities. Indianapolis, IN.

Answers to the Learning Assessment:

1. T
2. F
3. F
4. T
5. F

Index

Partnering for Recovery in Mental Health: A Practical Guide to Person-Centered Planning, First Edition.
Janis Tondora, Rebecca Miller, Mike Slade and Larry Davidson.
© 2014 John Wiley & Sons, Ltd. Published 2014 by John Wiley & Sons, Ltd.